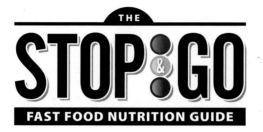

THE STOP & GO
FAST FOOD NUTRITION GUIDE

By Steven G. Aldana, PhD

MAPLE
MOUNTAIN
PRESS

The Stop & Go Fast Food Nutrition Guide

Nutrition data used in this guide has been provided by the individual
fast food restaurants.

Maple Mountain Press
935 East 900 North
Mapleton, UT 84664
phone: (801) 836-6388
email: info@maplemountainpress.com

ISBN 10: 0-9758828-4-8
ISBN 13: 978-0-9758828-4-9

Printed in the United States of America

Layout design and art direction by Brad Moulton
Maple Mountain Studio | www.maplemountainstudio.com

Table of Contents

Restaurants continued

Special thanks are given to Ann Bahr and the following experts for their critical review and excellent guidance. This guide could not have been possible without their input.

Marci Anderson, RD
Desiree Backman, Dr PH, MS, RD
Brian Becker, MD
Jennie Brand-Miller, PhD
T. Colin Campbell, PhD
Rebecca Vinton-Dorn, MA
Roger L. Greenlaw, MD, FACG, ABHM
Connie Guttersen, PhD, RD
Aaron Hardy, MS
Shereen Jegtvig
David L. Katz, MD, MPH, FACPM, FACP
Patty Kulbeth, RD
Susan McGreevy, MEd, CHES
Larry T. Tucker, PhD
Andrew Weil, MD

Fast food is awesome. You pull up in your car, speak into a microphone and in less than 30 seconds you are eating hot, tasty, inexpensive food. Fast food is any ready-to-eat food purchased and eaten away from home, including food from restaurants and convenience stores. Fast food is an American original; it was invented here. It reflects American attitudes and culture in that it embodies everything we value: it is tasty, convenient, inexpensive, and, most importantly, fast. Other factors in the popularity of fast food are that there is no preparation required before meals and no dishes to clean afterwards. Fast food is so popular, in fact, that today almost half of our food dollars are spent on fast foods.[1]

If you really care about your health, you know that avoiding tobacco, exercising regularly, and eating healthy foods are necessary. But is it possible to eat fast food and still be healthy? It is if you order the right kinds of fast food, and this guide will show you how to do it. By following three easy rules, you can eat out and still eat healthy. Before you turn to see if your favorite fast food items are healthy, however, you should read this introduction. It will explain why you should really care about choosing healthy fast foods, and it will help you understand how the guide was put together.

It is impossible to have a guide that everyone agrees with because people have different perspectives and ideas about what is and is not healthy. However, this guide was developed with the best science available, and it was carefully reviewed by a national panel of nutrition experts. This is not the only fast food guide available, but it represents the most comprehensive collection of nutritional data for fast food restaurants across the United States. It will help you navigate the fast food maze and make food choices that actually contribute to good health, not chronic disease.

If fast food is so much a part of our American culture, why do we need a fast food guide?

As a population, Americans have more body fat now than any other population at any time in human history. That's right. There has never been a population in world history that has had more body fat than Americans do right now. The most recent data from the Centers for Disease Control shows that 71% of men in the United States are overweight or obese,[2] just over 62% of women are overweight or obese, and children and adolescents are not immune. These two youngest groups in the American population have experienced the greatest increases in body fat of the past 20 years. Americans also have more type II diabetes than at any other time in history. Excessive body weight and diabetes cause many chronic diseases and will likely shorten the average lifespan in the United States by two to five years.[3] Consequently, this may be the first time in the past century that children will die at a younger age than their parents. So what does any of this have to do with fast food?

Despite great taste, low cost, and convenience, there is a darker, less desirable side of fast food. Much of the fast food Americans eat does not contribute to a healthy weight, and most of it may actually cause chronic diseases like heart disease, cancer, diabetes, and many others.

Here's the Proof

When you compare people who eat a lot of fast food with people who don't, there are several differences between the two groups. Fast food eaters consume more dietary fat and saturated fat. They also have more body fat, and they eat fewer fruits and vegetables.[4] Studies have shown this to be true for children, Black and White adolescent girls, college-aged adults, and middle-aged adults.[5-7] One study that took 15 years to complete showed that eating fast food was associated with diabetes and weight gain.[8]

It also seems that if you live near a lot of fast food restaurants, you are likely to eat more fast foods. A study in Ontario, Canada, found that people who lived near a lot of fast food restaurants were more likely to have heart disease and even premature death.[9] Another study revealed a correlation between the number of fast food restaurants per square mile and obesity in the 48 contiguous states: the states with the most fast food restaurants per square mile also had the highest rates of obesity.[10] Researchers in New Zealand gathered information from 1,300 children and found a direct relationship between asthma and the number of hamburgers children ate: those who ate the most hamburgers had the most asthma.[11]

The bad side of fast food is not just a problem for American citizens. Hispanic and Asian-American adolescents who have recently immigrated to the United States quickly assimilate American culture. Within one year after arriving in the United States, many immigrants exercise less and start to eat more fast foods—typical American behaviors that lead to obesity and chronic disease.[12] They learn to live like Americans and they will die like Americans.

But Wait, It Gets Worse

What the results of this research revealed is bad, but the problems with eating most fast food are much worse. Researchers from around the world have been carefully studying what people eat and what diseases they get later in life. Using very large research studies, they have been able to identify diets that either contribute to good health or are associated with chronic diseases.

There are two diet patterns that appear to either cause or prevent chronic diseases. The diet pattern associated with the best health is called the prudent diet. The diet that is the most unhealthy is called the Western diet. "Western" refers to countries that have become Westernized—basically the industrialized nations of the world that are a lot like America. This Western diet is fairly typical of what many Americans eat, especially those who eat a lot of fast food. Typical foods of the Western diet include the following:

Stop & Go **Fast Food Nutrition Guide**

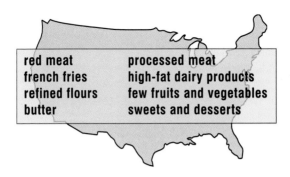

red meat   processed meat
french fries   high-fat dairy products
refined flours few fruits and vegetables
butter   sweets and desserts

The prudent diet, on the other hand, is quite different. The pyramid below shows what the prudent diet looks like. For many Americans, it may look nothing like what they normally eat.

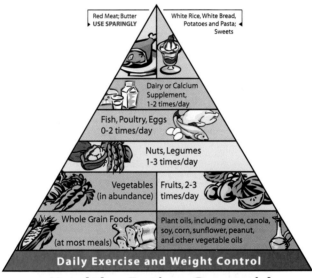

Healthy Eating Pyramid

The Prudent Diet Pattern

http://www.hsph.harvard.edu/nutritionsource - Used with permission.

The top of the pyramid suggests that foods shown here should be eaten sparingly. Notice that many of the foods listed there are part of the Western diet. The prudent diet is based on healthy plant oils, whole grains, fruits and vegetables, nuts and legumes (beans), fish, poultry, and eggs. Which of these patterns best describes your diet? Do you follow a prudent diet or a Western diet?

Through large studies with hundreds of thousands of participants, researchers determined that if you follow a prudent diet, you lower your risk of developing diabetes by 16%, but if you follow a Western diet, your risk of developing diabetes increases by 59%.[13,14] The prudent diet is associated with a 34% decrease in risk of heart disease, and the Western diet was linked with a 64% increase in heart disease risk.[15-17] These two diet patterns were even associated with other chronic diseases like colon cancer[18] and strokes.[19] Those who eat a prudent diet reduce their risk of chronic disease; those who eat a Western diet significantly increase their risk.

While these two diet patterns were accurate in describing who might and who might not get diabetes, heart disease, stroke, and colon cancer, not all chronic diseases are related to these two diet patterns. When the same patterns were used to determine who might get breast or prostate cancer, there was no difference between the two.[20,21] However, a prudent diet does appear to help breast cancer survivors avoid other causes of death not associated with the cancer.[22]

Individuals who eat typical American fast food are eating a Western diet. Most fast food contains a lot of red and processed meats, white flour, butter, and other high-fat dairy products. French fries and sweets and desserts are very popular fast foods. In fact, fast food is a Western diet. That means that most fast food is actually causing many of the chronic diseases most Americans suffer from, including obesity.

There's More . . .

Ahhh . . . the smell of fresh pastries, cookies, and cakes. Who can resist? Almost all foods that are commercially fried are fried in trans fats. We've been hearing a lot about trans fats in the news, and now all packaged foods are required to display information about trans fat content. Trans fats are plant oils that are altered in a process called hydrogenation. In this process, healthy plant oils are heated to about 400 degrees and hydrogen gas and a metal catalyst are added. This makes the vegetable oil accept additional hydrogen atoms and—presto!—what used to be a healthy vegetable oil is now a saturated fat with special properties. It can be used to fry food over and over again without going rancid, and it has a very long shelf life. Almost all fast food restaurants use trans fats for frying because it is relatively inexpensive. Furthermore, trans fats have a texture most people like. For example, margarine, which is made mostly from trans fats, is softer than real butter and easier to work with, and pie crusts, crackers, and croissants are flakier when made with trans fats.

This is where science once again shows us some warning signs. There have been 16 studies that have looked at links between trans fats and chronic disease.[23] All but 2 of the 16 studies showed that consuming trans fats is probably harmful. The prudent diet pyramid shows that healthy plant oils like olive, peanut, and soybean oil should be part of a healthy diet. These oils are high in poly- and monounsaturated fats. They are actually good for you because they improve your blood cholesterol. Trans fats, on the other hand, dramatically increase your risk of heart disease because they make cholesterol worse. In fact, trans fats are thought to be 10 times worse than saturated fats. If you are going to eat fast foods, you are going to dramatically increase your risk of heart attack and stroke because most fast foods contain a lot of trans fats.

This research is so convincing that the latest U.S. government nutrition recommendations encourage Americans to keep the intake of trans fats as low as possible. The minimum amount of trans fats a person can consume and not increase risk is zero.

Dr. Walter Willett, chair of the department of nutrition at the Harvard School of Public Health, recently stated,

> "In Europe [food companies] hired chemists and took trans fats out.... In the United States, they hired lawyers and public relations people. No one doubted trans fats have adverse affects on health, and still companies were not taking it out."

Any fast food that is deep fried is likely to be fried in trans fats. As you will see in this guide, some fast food companies no longer use trans fats, but most still do. If the safe recommended amount of trans fats is zero, should you eat a large order of McDonald's french fries if it contains 8 grams of trans fats? What about the yummy doughnuts at Krispy Kreme? They are fried in trans fats, and in this guide they are all coded red to help remind you to avoid eating them.

Since fast food is purchased hot, it is not required to have a nutrition label and you will never really know about the trans fat content. Think of all the fried foods in American fare: french fries, onion rings, corn dogs, popcorn, seafood, chips, and, oooh, those bakery goods. Maple bars, doughnuts, croissants, éclairs—all of them are either made with trans fats or are deep fried in trans fats. The only way you would know would be if you were to see a list of the ingredients or to read the label on the oil being used. You won't see the words "trans fats" in the ingredients. If a food has trans fats, it will be listed as partially hydrogenated oil, the technical term for trans fats.

According to a survey conducted by the Center for Science in the Public Interest (CSPI), the biggest restaurant chains still fry french fries, chicken nuggets, and other foods in trans fats.[24] The CSPI survey, which included 38 major food manufacturers, 100 restaurant chains, and 25 supermarket chains, revealed many interesting insights into the fast food industry. For example, while several major restaurant chains, including Taco Bell and Pizza Hut, are testing healthier oils, only a few chains have already taken action to actually use healthier oils.

The Good Guys

- Au Bon Pain, a 220-location café chain based in Boston, has eliminated trans fat from all of its cookies, bagels, and muffins, and is now using a nonhydrogenated margarine.
- Jason's Deli, a 137-outlet sandwich and salad chain, has stopped using partially hydrogenated oils in all of its products.
- Panera Bread, a 773-outlet café chain that was formerly part of Au Bon Pain, is in the process of replacing all partially hydrogenated oils and plans to be trans fat–free by year's end.
- California Pizza Kitchen has removed trans fat from deep-fried foods and is working on eliminating it from all other foods.
- In 2005 Ruby Tuesday, with some 700 table-service restaurants around the country, began deep-frying in heart-healthy canola oil.
- Chick-fil-A fries in peanut oil in its outlets.

The Bad Guys

- Starbucks, ice-cream chain Friendly's, and fried-chicken chain Popeyes indicated they had no plans to remove or reduce trans fat in their foods.
- Meals at other restaurants also are loaded with trans fat. KFC's chicken pot pie contains 14 grams of trans, and Taco Bell's Nachos BellGrande has 7 grams.

From http://www.cspinet.org/new/pdf/trans_report.pdf

In 2002, McDonald's promised to reduce and ultimately eliminate the trans fat in its cooking oil, but in 2003 it quietly backed away from this effort. McDonald's lost a lawsuit related to this matter and was ordered to give $7 million to the American Heart Association to be used to educate the public about the dangers of trans fats. McDonald's has reformulated its Chicken McNuggets and a few other products to have a little less trans fat, but its fried foods are still very high in trans fats. A McDonald's meal that includes a five-piece Chicken Selects Breast Strips order and a medium order of french fries has about 9.5 grams of trans fats. A piece of baked apple pie at McDonald's has 5 grams. Isn't it strange that McDonald's outlets in Australia, Denmark, and Israel all fry in trans fat free oil but Americans still get the trans fats?

So What's the Big Deal?

If Americans would reduce the amount of trans fats they are currently eating, it is estimated that 30,000 to 100,000 heart disease deaths would be prevented every year.[25] That would provide a bigger improvement in public health than just about any other medical breakthrough in the past 100 years!

But this guide isn't just about trans fats. Fruits and vegetables and whole grains are also very important. A review of the science reveals that Americans who increase their fruit and vegetable consumption from two servings per day to five or more can cut their risk of many cancers in half.[26]

Obviously, scientists haven't answered all the nutrition questions, but they have discovered enough information to help Americans prevent, arrest, and even reverse most chronic diseases. All it takes is good nutrition, regular physical activity, and avoiding tobacco use.

Be Careful What You Order

A quick look at many of the foods in this guide reveals a few surprises. First of all, the calorie content of some of America's fast food is shocking. Let's put this into perspective. The average person weighs 156 pounds. When walking at a pace of 3 miles per hour, that person expends about 5.1 calories per minute. Say you decide to have dinner at Chili's, and for a starter you order the Awesome Blossom. This "starter" contains 2,710 calories. If you were the average person, you would have to walk 27 miles to burn off all the calories you just ate and it would take you about 9 hours of walking to do it. The table below shows some other fast food calorie counts that you might find enlightening.

	Calories	Miles you would need to walk to burn off these calories	How long you have to walk
Appetizer/Starters			
Chili's Awesome Blossom	2,710	27 miles	9 hours
Denny's Mini burgers w/onion rings	2,044	20 miles	7 hours
Entrées			
McDonald's hamburger	260	3 miles	1 hour
McDonald's Big Mac	560	5 miles	2 hours
Romano's Macaroni Grill Spaghetti & Meatballs dinner	2,270	22 miles	7 hours
Nathan's Famous Seafood Sampler	3,379	33 miles	11 hours
Shoney's Deluxe Pancake Plate	1,609	16 miles	5 hours
Lone Star Steakhouse Lone Star Wings	1,759	17 miles	6 hours
O'Charley's chicken tenders dinner	1,359	13 miles	4 hours
Dessert			
Romano's Macaroni Grill New York cheesecake with caramel fudge sauce	1,760	17 miles	6 hours

How This Guide Was Developed

To help you make healthy fast food choices, almost 3,500 different foods have been color coded after an exhaustive process used to determine if a food should be red, yellow, or green. We contacted the 200 largest fast food companies in America and requested nutrition information about each of their menu items. Companies are not required by law to provide the nutrition information for the foods they sell—this is strictly voluntary—and most companies do not have any nutrition information about their foods. Still, we were able to gather nutrition information from 68 restaurants.

The available nutrition information on these fast foods was then entered into a large database and specifically designed computer programs identified foods that had any of the following characteristics:

More than 1 gram of trans fat per serving
More than 10 grams of saturated fat per serving
More than 125 milligrams of cholesterol per serving
More than 1,250 milligrams of sodium per serving

There is nothing magical about these criteria, except that some of them represent half the daily value for an average person. In other words, if a single fast food serving had more than half the amount of saturated fat, cholesterol, or sodium that a person should have in a single day, it was identified. Foods that contained lots of trans fats and little fiber were also identified. Any food that met none or just one of these criteria started off as green. Any food that met two of the criteria was initially coded yellow and any food that met three or more of the criteria was coded red. (Kind of like three strikes and you're out.)

There is an easier way to think about this coding. By using the prudent diet pyramid, a similar type of coding could be done. The pyramid shown below shows how foods could be coded according to where they are located on the pyramid. Healthy green-coded foods would be those at the bottom of the pyramid; yellow toward the middle; and red foods, which should be eaten sparingly, are located at the top.

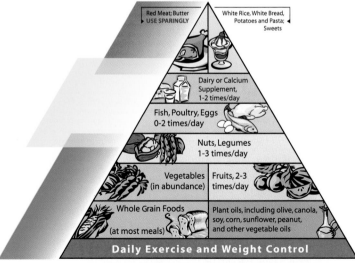

Healthy Eating Pyramid

Adapted from http://www.hsph.harvard.edu/nutritionsource

A further set of rules was also established to help in the coding process:

- Any food that had more than 1 gram of trans fat was automatically coded red.
- Foods that contained processed meats (meats like pepperoni, bacon, sausage, bologna, and hot dogs) or more than the recommended serving of red meat were also coded red.
- Foods that were initially coded as yellow and had amounts of sodium, saturated fat, or cholesterol that were not extremely high but were leaning in that direction, were moved to red.

To ensure consistent coding, the entire fast food dataset was reevaluated and coded three times. To further classify the foods, a distinguished panel of national nutrition and health promotion experts from across the United States was organized. These experts reviewed the entire process and suggested changes in the way the foods were coded. The experts are listed in the acknowledgments section. A final analysis shows that 33% of the foods in this guide are coded green, 20% are coded yellow, and 47% are coded red.

Fast Food and Good Health with Three Easy Rules

How can you make the best choices when you're eating fast food? This guide codes food as red, yellow, or green, depending on how healthy they are or not. Here are three easy rules to help you use this system to make healthy fast food choices:

Rule #1: Avoid the red foods.
Rule #2: Go easy on the yellow foods.
Rule #3: Eat healthy with the green foods.

Red foods = Hit the brakes!

There are many factors that result in a red code for a food. The number one factor why many foods receive a red code is that they contain more than one gram of trans fat. Lots of foods are coded red because they have more than one gram of trans fat content. Almost all of the foods at Taco Bell, for example, are coded red because they contain large amounts of trans fats. Many restaurants do not report the trans fat content of their foods—indicated in the table as not available (NA)—leading us to believe that they are still frying in trans fats (see Popeyes Chicken & Biscuits, for example). Consequently, they are coded red.

French fries are coded red because almost all restaurants fry them in trans fats. Any company that switches to healthier oils could instantly get a change in its food colors. For example, the In-N-Out burger chain located in California, Nevada, and Arizona fries in 100% cottonseed oil that is not hydrogenated. It's trans fat free and better for you, but french fries should still be a small part of a healthy diet. In-N-Out Burger's french fries get a green code! The only other restaurant that uses healthy oils for frying is Chick-fil-A, which has mostly green-coded foods because they fry in peanut oil.

As you will read later, foods fried in healthy oils can actually be good for you. Panda Express does not use trans fats in any of its fried food and is the only restaurant in this entire guide that receives a green code for all of its foods.

On the other hand, doughnut producers Krispy Kreme and Dunkin' Donuts have only red-coded foods because they are all made with trans fats. One doughnut can have as much as 5 grams of trans fats! Doughnuts are a wonderful treat, but they are also a food that should be eaten very sparingly if you care about good health.

Foods made with processed meats or that have a large serving of red meat are also coded red. A McDonald's regular hamburger—the small one that has just a squirt of ketchup, mustard, and a pickle—is actually coded green. It contains a small serving of red meat and not very many calories. A Big Mac, on the other hand, is a real heavy hitter with half the saturated fat for a whole day and trans fats. How would you color code a Pizza Hut Meat Lover's pizza? Even though it doesn't contain any trans fats, it gets a red in this guide because one slice contains a lot of saturated fat, sodium, and processed meat.

Desserts typically offered at restaurants are coded red because they generally contain a lot of calories, saturated fat, refined flour, and sugars. Therefore, desserts should be an occasional treat, not foods we eat often.

Yellow foods = Exercise caution!

What about a pizza that doesn't contain any processed meat? Your basic cheese pizza gets a yellow code. Although it doesn't contain trans fats or processed meat, it also doesn't contain any vegetables or whole grains. It's kind of in the middle. That's what yellow foods are like. They aren't good enough to be coded green or bad enough to deserve being branded red. Some yellow foods include:
Cheese pizza
Sweet and sour chicken
A single taco or burrito
Frozen yogurt

Green foods = You're eatin' healthy!

Green foods are the best. To earn the green badge of honor, a food has to have certain qualities that make it part of a healthy daily diet. Obviously foods made with whole grains, fruits, vegetables, and healthy oils will be coded green. Green-coded foods include vegetable pizza, many sandwiches, salads, eggs, and entrées made with vegetables, such as vegetable stir-fry. Green foods are low in saturated and trans fats, they don't contain excessive amounts of sodium or cholesterol, and they are relatively low in calories compared to yellow and red foods. They are actually good for you and could be eaten every day. By choosing green foods, you can eat fast food and still eat healthy . . . the best of both worlds. Another way to identify green foods is to ask the question: Is this food close to its natural/original form? A salad, for example, contains foods close to their natural form. A Hostess Twinkie, on the other hand, leaves us to wonder what its natural form actually was. A baked potato is going to be coded green, but trans fat fried tater tots are going to be red. You get the idea.

Some Restaurants Are Healthier Than Others

As you will see in this guide, some fast food restaurants sell a lot of red foods. Others have a lot more healthy choices. Based on the types of foods a restaurant serves, it is possible to produce a short list of restaurants ranked from best to worst according to the color-coding of the food they sell. Counting up the number of green, yellow, and red foods sold by different restaurants shows that some restaurants offer healthier foods than others:

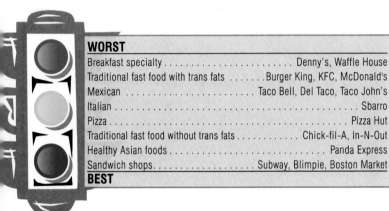

WORST

Breakfast specialty	Denny's, Waffle House
Traditional fast food with trans fats	Burger King, KFC, McDonald's
Mexican	Taco Bell, Del Taco, Taco John's
Italian	Sbarro
Pizza	Pizza Hut
Traditional fast food without trans fats	Chick-fil-A, In-N-Out
Healthy Asian foods	Panda Express
Sandwich shops	Subway, Blimpie, Boston Market

BEST

A Few Fast Food Marketing Tricks You Should Know About

Fast food restaurants are really designed and created to do one thing—sell as much food as possible. It doesn't matter if people eat the food because the main goal is to sell food. To do this, food venders use time-tested methods to get each customer to buy as much food as possible. No one likes to waste food, so when we do purchase a little extra food, the only responsible thing to do is eat it. Don't fall prey to these tricks and you won't feel obligated to eat all the food you buy.

Up-selling

Would you like egg rolls with that order? Do you want me to super size your meal? Would you like to make that a combo meal? These are all questions you might be asked next time you order fast food. It's called up-selling. You've already ordered what you want, you're ready to pay, and the person working at the counter asks you an up-sell question. The idea is to get as much money out of you as possible by selling you more food—food that you may or may not want or need. McDonald's super-sizing items and selling foods as part of a combo meal are examples of effective ways fast food restaurants get just a little more out of you each time you visit. Don't fall for it! Decide what you want before you get to the counter (hopefully picking green-coded foods) and don't buy any more food, no matter how hard the employee tries to sell it to you.

What smells so good?

Have you ever walked past a restaurant and smelled barbeque, fresh bread, or hot pastries? Most food producers don't purposely fill the air with the smells of their foods, but some do. By setting up a barbeque grill outside or venting kitchen grill smoke to the outside, they are advertising their food to the olfactory senses of the masses. If you're hungry and you've got a little extra cash, you may end up as their next customer.

It's all about the playground

Forget about the food; the kids will want to play at the fast food playground. Slides, treehouses, ball pits, and swings are attractive to small children, and playgrounds and even arcades have become common features in fast food restaurants. Restaurants know parents want to watch their kids play in a relatively confined space while they eat in peace. The combination of food and an attraction for the kids is a powerful marketing ploy. Unfortunately, the food often doesn't contribute to good health.

Forget the food, I want the toy!

The fast food industry excels at getting to us through our kids, and the kid's meal is another powerful fast food marketing tactic. Hollywood and the fast food industry have collaborated to create a marriage between fast food and movie marketing that results in children begging for the next plastic action hero that comes with fast food they might or might not eat. After all, what could be better than sharing a deep-fried meal with Luke Skywalker?

It's all in a name

Restaurant owners are pros at getting us to buy and eat. If a menu has chocolate cake, it won't sell well. But if the same menu has Black Forest Double-Chocolate Cake, the customer will be much more likely to purchase it and much more likely to approve of the taste. Why would Romano's Macaroni Grill sell cheesecake when it can sell New York cheesecake with caramel fudge sauce? Just the name of the food can impact sales and customer satisfaction.[27] Don't be swayed too much by the names. Listen to your body and let your stomach tell you when you are full.

Fast Food Is Only Part of the Problem

It wouldn't be fair to place all of the blame for America's poor health on the fast food industry. There are several reasons why Americans are not as healthy as they should be. Regardless of what we eat, we eat too much. We don't get much exercise, and we have a culture and environment that discourage healthy eating and regular physical activity. This guide is designed to help you still enjoy fast food by selecting fast foods that are actually good for you. When combined with regular exercise, you will be well on your way to good health and a healthy body weight.

When all is said and done, everyone eats fast foods. Good health is just a matter of sorting through and eating the right ones.

Fast food restaurants are always changing. For the latest restaurant updates go to:

www.WellSteps.com

REFERENCES

1. Lin B, Guthrie J, Frazao E. Nutrient contribution of food away from home. In: America's Eating Habits: Changes and Consequences, 1999, pages 213–242. U.S. Department of Agriculture, Economic Research Service, Washington, D.C. Agriculture Information Bulletin No. 750.

2. Ogden CL, Carroll MD, Curtin LR, McDowell MA, Tabak CJ, Flegal KM, Prevalence of Overweight and Obesity in the United States, 1999–2004, JAMA. 2006;295:1549-1555.

3. Olshansky SJ, Passaro DJ, Hershow RC, Layden J, Carnes BA, Brody J, Hayflick L, Butler RN, Allison DB, Ludwig DS. A potential decline in life expectancy in the United States in the 21st century. N Engl J Med. 2005 Mar 17;352(11):1138-45.

4. Jeffery RW, Baxter J, McGuire M, Linde J.Are fast food restaurants an environmental risk factor for obesity? Int J Behav Nutr Phys Act. 2006 Jan 25;3:2.

5. Schmidt M, Affenito SG, Striegel-Moore R, Khoury PR, Barton B, Crawford P, Kronsberg S, Schreiber G, Obarzanek E, Daniels S. Fast-food intake and diet quality in black and white girls: the National Heart, Lung, and Blood Institute Growth and Health Study. Arch Pediatr Adolesc Med. 2005 Jul;159(7):626-31.

6. Bowman SA, Vinyard BT. Fast food consumption of U.S. adults: impact on energy and nutrient intakes and overweight status. J Am Coll Nutr. 2004 Apr;23(2):163-8.

7. Bowman SA, Gortmaker SL, Ebbeling CB, Pereira MA, Ludwig DS.Effects of fast-food consumption on energy intake and diet quality among children in a national household survey. Pediatrics. 2004 Jan;113(1 Pt 1):112-8.

8. Pereira MA, Kartashov AI, Ebbeling CB, Van Horn L, Slattery ML, Jacobs DR Jr, Ludwig DS. Fast-food habits, weight gain, and insulin resistance (the CARDIA study):15-year prospective analysis. Lancet. 2005 Jan 1- 7;365(9453):36-42.

9. Alter DA, Eny K. The relationship between the supply of fast-food chains and cardiovascular outcomes. Can J Public Health. 2005 May-Jun;96(3):173-7.

10. Maddock J. The relationship between obesity and the prevalence of fast food restaurants: state-level analysis. Am J Health Promot. 2004 Nov-Dec;19(2):137-43.

11. Wickens K, Barry D, Friezema A, Rhodius R, Bone N, Purdie G, Crane J. Fast foods - are they a risk factor for asthma? Allergy. 2005 Dec;60(12):1537-41.

12. Unger JB, Reynolds K, Shakib S, Spruijt-Metz D, Sun P, Johnson CA. Acculturation, physical activity, and fast-food consumption among Asian-American and Hispanic adolescents. J Community Health. 2004 Dec;29(6):467-81.

13. van Dam RM, Rimm EB, Willett WC, Stampfer MJ, Hu FB. Dietary patterns and risk for type 2 diabetes mellitus in U.S. men. Ann Intern Med. 2002 Feb 5;136(3):201–9.

14. Hu FB, Manson JE, Stampfer MJ, Colditz G, Liu S, Solomon CG, Willett WC. Diet, lifestyle, and the risk of type 2 diabetes mellitus in women. N Engl J Med. 2001 Sep 13;345(11):790–7.

15. Fung TT, Willett WC, Stampfer MJ, Manson JE, Hu FB. Dietary patterns and the risk of coronary heart disease in women. Arch Intern Med. 2001 Aug 13-27;161(15):1857–62.

16. Schulze MB, Hu FB. Dietary patterns and risk of hypertension, type 2 diabetes mellitus, and coronary heart disease. Curr Atheroscler Rep. 2002 Nov;4(6):462–7.

17. Millen BE, Quatromoni PA, Nam BH, O'Horo CE, Polak JF, Wolf PA, D'Agostino RB; Framingham Nutrition Studies. Dietary patterns, smoking, and subclinical heart disease in women: opportunities for primary prevention from the Framingham Nutrition Studies. J Am Diet Assoc. 2004 Feb;104(2):208–14.

18. Terry P, Hu FB, Hansen H, Wolk A. Prospective study of major dietary patterns and colorectal cancer risk in women. Am J Epidemiol. 2001 Dec 15;154(12):1143–9.

19. Ding EL, Mozaffarian D. Optimal dietary habits for the prevention of stroke. Semin Neurol. 2006 Feb;26(1):11-23.

20. Terry P, Suzuki R, Hu FB, Wolk A. A prospective study of major dietary patterns and the risk of breast cancer. Cancer Epidemiol Biomarkers Prev. 2001 Dec;10(12):1281–5.

21. Wu K, Hu FB, Willett WC, Giovannucci E. Dietary patterns and risk of prostate cancer in U.S. men. Cancer Epidemiol Biomarkers Prev. 2006 Jan;15(1):167-71.

22. Kroenke CH, Fung TT, Hu FB, Holmes MD. Dietary patterns and survival after breast cancer diagnosis. J Clin Oncol. 2005 Dec 20;23(36):9295-303.

23. Stender S, Dyerberg J. Influence of trans fatty acids on health. Ann Nutr Metab. 2004;48(2):61-6. Epub 2003 Dec 16.

24. Center for Science in the Public Interest, 2005 http://www.cspinet.org/new/ pdf/trans_report.pdf

25, Willett, Walter, Personal communication, 2006

26. Block G, Patterson B, and Subar A. Fruit, vegetables, and cancer prevention: A review of epidemiological evidence. Nutr and Cancer. 1992; 18:1–29.

27. Wansink B, Painter JM, Ittersum K, Descriptive Menu Labels Effect on Sales, Cornell Hotel and Restaurant Administrative Quarterly, 2001,42:6 December, 68-72.

Most fast food restaurants offer the same beverages. To simplify the menu lists in this section of the guide, beverage information has been consolidated in the list below. Also, throughout the menu lists space has been provided for you to make notes. As you eat at different fast food restaurants, write down what you do and don't like about your eating experience. Use your notes to make your next fast food meal even healthier!

Drinks

	Serving	Calories	Total fat (gm)	Saturated fat (gm)	Trans fats (gm)	Cholesterol (mg)	Sodium (mg)	Carbs (gm)
Milk								
Whole	1 cup	146	8	5	0	24	98	12
2%	1 cup	122	5	3	0	20	100	12
1%	1 cup	102	2	2	0	12	107	12
Skim or Non-Fat	1 cup	83	0	0	0	5	103	12
Other Drinks								
100% Fruit Juices	1 cup	110	0	0	0	0	20	30
Bottled Water	1 bottle	0	0	0	0	0	0	0
Fountain Drinks								
A&W Diet Root Beer	15 fl. oz.	0	0	0	0	0	40	0
A&W Root Beer	15 fl. oz.	220	0	0	0	0	40	60
Barq's Root Beer	16 fl. oz.	147	0	0	0	0	32	60
Caffeine Free Diet Coke	16 fl. oz.	0	0	0	0	0	13	0
Cherry Coca-Cola	16 fl. oz.	137	0	0	0	0	5	56
Coca-Cola Classic	16 fl. oz.	131	0	0	0	0	8	54
Diet Caffeine Free Pepsi	16 fl. oz.	0	0	0	0	0	40	0
Diet Coke	16 fl. oz.	1	0	0	0	0	13	0
Diet Dr. Pepper	16 fl. oz.	0	0	0	0	0	48	0
Diet Mountain Dew	16 fl. oz.	0	0	0	0	0	40	0
Diet Pepsi	16 fl. oz.	0	0	0	0	0	40	0
Dr. Pepper	16 fl. oz.	132	0	0	0	0	48	52
Fanta Orange	16 fl. oz.	148	0	0	0	0	11	70
Hi-C Flashin' Fruit Punch	16 fl. oz.	137	0	0	0	0	12	56
Hi-C Orange Lavaburst	16 fl. oz.	147	0	0	0	0	0	60
Lipton Brisk (sweetened)	16 fl. oz.	92	0	0	0	0	40	44
Lipton Brisk (unsweetened)	16 fl. oz.	0	0	0	0	0	40	0
Lipton Brisk Lemonade	16 fl. oz.	132	0	0	0	0	119	44
Lipton Brisk Raspberry	16 fl. oz.	106	0	0	0	0	0	46
Mello Yello	16 fl. oz.	140	0	0	0	0	11	64
Minute Maid Lemonade	16 fl. oz.	128	0	0	0	0	54	56
Minute Maid Light Lemonade	16 fl. oz.	7	0	0	0	0	7	10
Minute Maid Orange	16 fl. oz.	140	0	0	0	0	0	54
Mountain Dew	16 fl. oz.	145	0	0	0	0	46	62
Mountain Dew Code Red	16 fl. oz.	145	0	0	0	0	46	62
Mug Root Beer	16 fl. oz.	132	0	0	0	0	40	58

Drinks Continued

Fountain Drinks continued

	Serving	Calories	Total fat (gm)	Saturated fat (gm)	Trans fats (gm)	Cholesterol (mg)	Sodium (mg)	Carbs (gm)
Nestea Iced Tea (sweetened)	16 fl. oz.	82	0	0	0	0	18	34
Nestea Iced Tea (unsweetened)	16 fl. oz.	1	0	0	0	0	18	0
Nestea Raspberry Iced Tea	16 fl. oz.	103	0	0	0	0	12	42
Pepsi	16 fl. oz.	132	0	0	0	0	33	62
Pibb Xtra	16 fl. oz.	128	0	0	0	0	18	52
POWERade Mountain Blast	16 fl. oz.	95	0	0	0	0	20	34
Sierra Mist	16 fl. oz.	132	0	0	0	0	33	52
Sierra Mist Free	16 fl. oz.	0	0	0	0	0	33	0
Slice	16 fl. oz.	145	0	0	0	0	46	54
Sprite	16 fl. oz.	128	0	0	0	0	29	52
Squirt	16 fl. oz.	132	0	0	0	0	22	54
Wild Cherry Pepsi	16 fl. oz.	145	0	0	0	0	33	56

A & W®

Sandwiches & Strips

	Serving	Calories	Total fat (gm)	Saturated fat (gm)	Trans fats (gm)	Cholesterol (mg)	Sodium (mg)	Carbs (gm)
Hamburger	1 item	460	22	8	3	75	690	NA
Cheeseburger	1 item	500	24	9	3	90	870	NA
Deluxe Hamburger	1 item	460	26	7	2.5	65	840	NA
Deluxe Cheeseburger	1 item	510	28	8	2.5	80	1020	NA
Deluxe Double Cheeseburger	1 item	720	42	15	2.5	150	1370	46
Deluxe Bacon Cheeseburger	1 item	570	33	10	2.5	90	1200	41
Deluxe Bacon Double Cheeseburger	1 item	800	48	17	2.5	165	1600	47
Papa Burger	1 item	720	42	15	4	145	1390	46
Grilled Chicken Sandwich	1 item	430	15	3.5	2	90	1080	34
Crispy Chicken Sandwich	1 item	580	25	5	3	65	1390	54
Chicken Strips	3 piece	500	29	5	2	55	1050	32

Hot Dogs & Coneys

	Serving	Calories	Total fat (gm)	Saturated fat (gm)	Trans fats (gm)	Cholesterol (mg)	Sodium (mg)	Carbs (gm)
Hot Dog (plain)	1 item	280	17	6	1	35	710	22
Cheese Dog	1 item	320	20	7	1	40	910	25
Coney Chili Dog	1 item	310	18	7	1	40	870	24
Coney Chili Cheese Dog	1 item	350	21	8	1	45	1070	27

Side Items

	Serving	Calories	Total fat (gm)	Saturated fat (gm)	Trans fats (gm)	Cholesterol (mg)	Sodium (mg)	Carbs (gm)
Kid's Fries	4 oz.	310	13	4	4	0	460	45
French Fries	5.5 oz.	430	18	5	6	0	640	61
Chili Fries	6 oz.	370	16	5	4	10	780	49
Cheese Fries	6 oz.	380	19	5	4	5	870	50
Chili/Cheese Fries	7 oz.	400	19	5	4	10	990	51
Onion Rings	4 oz.	350	17	4	7	5	720	45
Cheese Curds	1 item	570	40	21	1	105	1220	NA
Chili Bowl	1 item	190	6	2	0	20	640	22

Applebee's®

Does provides limited nutrition Information.

	Serving	Calories	Total fat (gm)	Saturated fat (gm)	Trans fats (gm)	Cholesterol (mg)	Sodium (mg)	Carbs (gm)
Tortilla Chicken Melt	1 item	480	13	NA	NA	NA	NA	NA
Onion Soup Au Gratin	1 item	150	8	NA	NA	NA	NA	NA
Italian Chicken & Portobello Sandwich	1 item	360	6	NA	NA	NA	NA	NA
Steak and Portobellos	1 item	330	10	NA	NA	NA	NA	NA
Cajun Lime Tilapia	1 item	310	6	NA	NA	NA	NA	NA
Southwest Cobb Salad	1 item	440	8	NA	NA	NA	NA	NA
Teriyaki Steak n' Shrimp Skewers	1 item	370	7	NA	NA	NA	NA	NA
Grilled Shrimp Skewer Salad	1 item	210	2	NA	NA	NA	NA	NA
Confetti Chicken	1 item	370	7	NA	NA	NA	NA	NA

Arby's®

Market Fresh Salads

	Serving	Calories	Total fat (gm)	Saturated fat (gm)	Trans fats (gm)	Cholesterol (mg)	Sodium (mg)	Carbs (gm)
Chicken Club Salad	366 g	487	25	8	0.5	178	1220	31
Martha's Vineyard Salad™	330 g	277	8	4	0	72	451	24
Santa Fe Salad™	365 g	477	21	6	0.5	53	1131	42
Santa Fe Salad™ w/ Grilled Chicken	350 g	283	9	4	0	72	521	21

Market Fresh Sandwiches & Wraps

	Serving	Calories	Total fat (gm)	Saturated fat (gm)	Trans fats (gm)	Cholesterol (mg)	Sodium (mg)	Carbs (gm)
Corned Beef Reuben Wrap	280 g	577	29	8	0.5	83	1721	42
Roast Turkey Reuben Wrap	280 g	581	27	6	0	94	1301	43
Roast Ham & Swiss	359 g	705	31	8	0.5	63	2103	75
Chicken Club Wrap	1 Wrap	680	38	14	NA	100	1800	NA
Southwest Chicken Wrap	1 Wrap	550	30	9	1	75	1690	42
Chicken Salad w/ Pecans	322 g	769	39	10	0	74	1240	79
Chicken Salad w/ Pecans Wrap	277 g	638	38	10	1	74	1199	48
Corned Beef Reuben	309 g	606	33	9	0.5	83	1849	55
Roast Beef & Swiss	339 g	777	41	13	1.5	89	1743	73
Roast Turkey & Swiss	359 g	725	30	8	0.5	91	1788	75
Roast Turkey Ranch & Bacon	382 g	834	38	11	0.5	109	2258	75
Roast Turkey Ranch & Bacon Wrap	317 g	700	37	11	1	109	2215	44
Roast Turkey Reuben	309 g	611	30	8	0.5	94	1429	56
Southwest Chicken Wrap	254 g	567	29	9	1	88	1451	42
Ultimate BLT	294 g	779	45	11	0.5	51	1571	75
Ultimate BLT Wrap	249 g	648	44	11	1	51	1530	45
Fish Sandwich	239 g	543	25	6	0	55	956	61
Chicken Salad Sandwich	1 item	770	38	9	NA	75	1240	79
Roast Ham & Swiss	1 Sandwich	700	31	7	0.5	85	2140	75

Arby's® Continued

Desserts & Shakes

	Serving	Calories	Total fat (gm)	Saturated fat (gm)	Trans fats (gm)	Cholesterol (mg)	Sodium (mg)	Carbs (gm)
Apple Turnover	128 g	377	16	5	6.5	0	201	65
Cherry Turnover	128 g	377	15	5	6	0	201	65
Chocolate Chip Cookie	45 g	202	10	4	2	15	213	26
Chocolate (regular)	397 g	510	13	8	0	35	360	83
Chocolate (large)	510 g	660	17	10	.5	45	450	110
Jamocha (regular)	397 g	500	13	8	0	35	390	66
Jamocha (large)	510 g	650	17	10	.5	45	510	83
Strawberry (regular)	397 g	500	13	8	0	35	360	81
Strawberry (large)	510 g	650	17	10	.5	45	460	107
Vanilla (regular)	397 g	500	13	8	0	35	370	66
Vanilla (large)	510 g	650	17	10	.5	45	470	83

Arby's Chicken Naturals

	Serving	Calories	Total fat (gm)	Saturated fat (gm)	Trans fats (gm)	Cholesterol (mg)	Sodium (mg)	Carbs (gm)
Popcorn Chicken - Large	184 g	531	26	6	1	59	1666	39
Popcorn Chicken Shakers	240 g	585	27	6	1	59	2795	51
Popcorn Chicken - Regular	126 g	365	18	4	0.5	40	1145	27
Chicken Bacon & Swiss - Crispy	214 g	624	29	7	0	68	1320	52
Chicken Bacon & Swiss - Grilled	209 g	462	17	4	0	25	1333	38
Chicken Cordon Bleu Sandwich - Crispy	243 g	650	31	6	0.5	74	1548	49
Chicken Cordon Bleu Sandwich - Grilled	238 g	488	19	4	0	32	1561	35
Chicken Fillet Sandwich - Crispy	238 g	576	30	5	0	52	901	50
Chicken Fillet Sandwich - Grilled	233 g	414	17	3	0	9	913	36
Chicken Tenders - 3 piece	131 g	379	18	3	0	42	1188	28
Chicken Tenders - 5 piece	218 g	630	31	5	0	70	1977	47

Arby's Toasted Subs

	Serving	Calories	Total fat (gm)	Saturated fat (gm)	Trans fats (gm)	Cholesterol (mg)	Sodium (mg)	Carbs (gm)
Classic Italian	379 g	828	46	13	0.5	89	2496	69
French Dip & Swiss	337 g	622	20	7	1.5	79	3397	68
Philly Beef	281 g	739	37	9	1	85	1881	64
Turkey Bacon Club	341 g	619	18	4	0	82	2052	65

Sides & Sidekickers

	Serving	Calories	Total fat (gm)	Saturated fat (gm)	Trans fats (gm)	Cholesterol (mg)	Sodium (mg)	Carbs (gm)
Cheddar Fries - Medium	170 g	465	28	6	2	2	1311	51
Curly Fries - Large	198 g	631	37	7	1	0	1476	73
Curly Fries - Medium	125 g	397	24	4	0	0	928	46
Curly Fries - Small	106 g	338	20	4	0	0	791	39
Homestyle Fries - Large	213 g	566	37	7	1	0	1029	82
Homestyle Fries - Medium	142 g	377	25	4	0.5	0	686	55
Homestyle Fries - Small	113 g	302	20	4	0.5	0	549	44
Jalapeno Bites® - Large (10)	220 g	611	43	18	1.5	56	1052	58
Jalapeno Bites® - Regular (5)	110 g	305	21	9	1	28	526	29

Arby's® Continued

Sides & Sidekickers continued

	Serving	Calories	Total fat (gm)	Saturated fat (gm)	Trans fats (gm)	Cholesterol (mg)	Sodium (mg)	Carbs (gm)
Loaded Potato Bites™ - Large (10)	224 g	707	44	14	1.5	27	1601	54
Loaded Potato Bites™ - Regular (5)	112 g	353	22	7	0.5	13	800	27
Mozzarella Sticks - Regular (4)	137 g	426	28	13	1	45	1370	38
Mozzarella Sticks - Large (8)	273 g	849	56	26	2	90	2730	76
Onion Petals - Large	283 g	828	57	9	1	2	831	70
Onion Petals - Regular	113 g	331	23	4	0	1	332	35
Potato Cakes (2)	100 g	246	18	4	1	0	391	26
Popcorn Chicken	Regular	365	18	4	1	40	1145	27
Southwest Egg Rolls	4 Pieces	225	7	2	2	27	390	29

Arby's Roast Beef Sandwiches & Melts

	Serving	Calories	Total fat (gm)	Saturated fat (gm)	Trans fats (gm)	Cholesterol (mg)	Sodium (mg)	Carbs (gm)
Junior Roast Beef	125 g	272	10	4	0	29	740	34
Arby's Melt	146 g	302	12	4	1	30	921	NA
Bacon Beef 'n Cheddar	212 g	521	27	9	1.5	64	1573	45
Beef 'n Cheddar	195 g	445	21	6	1.5	51	1274	45
Fish Sandwich	1 Sandwich	545	25	6	0	55	955	61
French Dip & Swiss	224 g	473	18	7	1	79	1679	38
Ham & Swiss Melt	138 g	275	6	2	0	27	1118	35
Large Roast Beef	281 g	547	28	12	1.5	102	1869	41
Medium Roast Beef	210 g	415	21	9	1	73	1379	41
Regular Roast Beef	154 g	320	14	5	0.5	44	953	34
Giant Roast Beef	1 Sandwich	450	19	9	1	75	1440	41
Super Roast Beef	1 Sandwich	440	19	7	2	45	1130	40
Big Montana	1 Sandwich	590	29	14	NA	115	2080	NA
Sourdough Ham Melt	165 g	380	13	3	0	31	1280	39
Sourdough Roast Beef Melt	166 g	355	14	5	1	30	1047	40
Swiss Melt	146 g	303	12	4	1	29	919	37
Chicken Bacon 'N Swiss	1 Sandwich	550	27	7	0	70	1640	52
Spicy Cajun Fish Sandwich	1 Sandwich	605	32	7	0	68	885	61
Roast Chicken Club	1 Sandwich	470	25	7	NA	65	1320	NA
BBQ Bacon 'n Jack	Sandwich	360	15	5	1	38	1175	42

Kid's Meal

	Serving	Calories	Total fat (gm)	Saturated fat (gm)	Trans fats (gm)	Cholesterol (mg)	Sodium (mg)	Carbs (gm)
Kids Meal - Junior Roast Beef	125 g	272	10	4	0	29	740	34
Fruit Cup	57 g	35	0	0	0	0	0	9
Market Fresh™ Mini Ham & Cheese Sandwich	112 g	228	5	1	0	23	916	28
Market Fresh™ Mini Turkey & Cheese Sandwich	112 g	235	4	1	0	33	798	28
Kids Meal - Chicken Tenders 2 pc.	100 g	289	14	2	0	32	907	21

Arby's® Continued

Breakfast

	Serving	Calories	Total fat (gm)	Saturated fat (gm)	Trans fats (gm)	Cholesterol (mg)	Sodium (mg)	Carbs (gm)
Bacon & Egg Croissant	120 g	337	22	10	0	187	651	23
Bacon Biscuit	95 g	340	21	6	0	13	1028	29
Bacon, Egg & Cheese Biscuit	158 g	461	28	8	0	169	1446	40
Bacon, Egg & Cheese Croissant	133 g	378	22	10	0	198	850	24
Bacon, Egg & Cheese Sourdough	173 g	437	16	5	0	174	1220	40
Bacon, Egg, & Cheese Wrap	193 g	515	29	8	0.5	165	1367	50
Biscuit - Plain	82 g	273	15	4	0	1	786	28
Blueberry Muffin	85 g	320	12	2	0	20	490	49
Chicken Biscuit	132 g	417	23	5	0	17	1240	39
Croissant	1 item	190	10	6	0	30	190	21
Egg & Cheese Sourdough	164 g	392	12	3	0	166	1058	40
French Toastix	124 g	312	13	2	0	0	492	44
Sausage, Egg & Cheese Biscuit	185 g	557	38	11	0	187	1579	30
Sausage, Egg & Cheese Sourdough	191 g	514	27	8	0	186	1232	40
Ham & Cheese Croissant	113 g	274	12	7	0	53	842	22
Ham Biscuit	125 g	316	17	4	0	13	1240	29
Ham, Egg & Cheese Biscuit	188 g	437	23	6	0	169	1658	31
Ham, Egg & Cheese Croissant	213 g	434	24	10	0	343	1282	25
Ham, Egg & Cheese Sourdough	296 g	679	35	11	0	354	2104	42
Ham, Egg, & Cheese Wrap	242 g	568	31	10	1	183	1929	51
Sausage & Egg Croissant	147 g	433	32	13	0	206	784	23
Sausage Biscuit	122 g	436	31	9	0	32	1160	28
Sausage Gravy Biscuit	238 g	961	68	14	0	12	3755	107
Sausage Patty	51 g	210	20	7	0	40	480	0
Sausage, Egg & Cheese Croissant	160 g	475	32	13	0	216	982	23
Sausage, Egg & Cheese Wrap	239 g	689	45	15	1	202	1849	50

T.J. Cinnamons

	Serving	Calories	Total fat (gm)	Saturated fat (gm)	Trans fats (gm)	Cholesterol (mg)	Sodium (mg)	Carbs (gm)
Chocolate Twist	71 g	250	12	4	0	5	110	34
Cinnamon Twist	71 g	260	14	5	4	5	190	33
Original Gourmet Cinnamon Roll®	149 g	507	10	4	0	7	373	73
Pecan Sticky Bun	184 g	688	22	5	0	7	420	91
Pecan Sticky Bun 4 Pack	738 g	2751	90	21	0	30	1678	363
TJ Cinnamons Mocha Chill®	354 g	306	7	4	0	29	214	48

Auntie Ann's®

Pretzels & More

	Serving	Calories	Total fat (gm)	Saturated fat (gm)	Trans fats (gm)	Cholesterol (mg)	Sodium (mg)	Carbs (gm)
Almond Pretzel	1 item	400	8	5	0	20	400	72
Almond Pretzel w/o Butter	1 item	350	1.5	0.5	0	0	390	72
Cinnamon Sugar Pretzel	1 item	450	9	5	0	25	430	83
Cinnamon Sugar Pretzel w/o Butter	1 item	350	2	0	0	0	410	74
Garlic Pretzel	1 item	350	4.5	2.5	0	10	850	68
Garlic Pretzel w/o butter	1 item	320	1	0	0	0	830	66
Glazin' Raisin Pretzel	1 item	510	4	2	0	10	480	107
Glazin' Raisin Pretzel w/o butter	1 item	470	0.5	0	0	0	460	104
Jalapeño Pretzel	1 item	310	4.5	2.5	0	10	940	59
Jalapeño Pretzel w/o butter	1 item	270	1	0	0	0	780	58
Original Pretzel	1 item	370	4	2	0	10	930	72
Original Pretzel w/o butter	1 item	340	1	0	0	0	900	72
Pretzel Dog	1 item	290	16	7	0.5	40	600	25
Sesame Pretzel	1 item	410	12	4	0	15	860	64
Sesame Pretzel w/o butter	1 item	350	6	1	0	0	840	63
Sour Cream & Onion Pretzel	1 item	340	5	3	0	10	930	66
Sour Cream & Onion Pretzel w/o butter	1 item	310	1	0	0	0	920	66
Stix - Cinnamon Sugar	1 item	300	6	3	0	17	287	NA
Stix - Cinnamon Sugar w/o butter	1 item	233	1	0	0	0	273	NA
Stix - Original	1 item	247	3	1	0	7	620	72
Stix - Original w/o butter	1 item	227	1	0	0	0	600	72
Whole Wheat Pretzel	1 item	370	4.5	1.5	0	10	1120	72
Whole Wheat Pretzel w/o butter	1 item	350	1.5	0	0	0	1100	72

Dutch Ice

	Serving	Calories	Total fat (gm)	Saturated fat (gm)	Trans fats (gm)	Cholesterol (mg)	Sodium (mg)	Carbs (gm)
Grape Dutch Ice	14 fl. oz.	180	0	0	0	0	20	43
Grape Dutch Ice	20 fl. oz.	260	0	0	0	0	30	62
Kiwi-Banana Dutch Ice	14 fl. oz.	190	0	0	0	0	30	44
Kiwi-Banana Dutch Ice	20 fl. oz.	270	0	0	0	0	40	63
Lemonade Dutch Ice	14 fl. oz.	315	0	0	0	0	0	53
Lemonade Dutch Ice	20 fl. oz.	450	0	0	0	0	0	95
Mocha Dutch Ice	14 fl. oz.	400	10	9	0	0	100	74
Mocha Dutch Ice	20 fl. oz.	570	15	12.5	0	0	150	105
Orange Crème Dutch Ice	14 fl. oz.	280	0	0	0	0	35	64
Orange Crème Dutch Ice	20 fl. oz.	400	0	0	0	0	50	92
Piña Colada Dutch Ice	14 fl. oz.	250	0	0	0	0	20	53
Piña Colada Dutch Ice	20 fl. oz.	535	0	0	0	0	30	125
Blue Raspberry Dutch Ice	14 fl. oz.	175	0	0	0	0	30	38
Blue Raspberry Dutch Ice	20 fl. oz.	250	0	0	0	0	40	55
Strawberry Dutch Ice	14 fl. oz.	220	0	0	0	0	40	50

Auntie Ann's®
Continued
Dutch Ice continued

	Serving	Calories	Total fat (gm)	Saturated fat (gm)	Trans fats (gm)	Cholesterol (mg)	Sodium (mg)	Carbs (gm)
Strawberry Dutch Ice	20 fl. oz.	315	0	0	0	0	60	72
Wild Cherry Dutch Ice	14 fl. oz.	230	0	0	0	0	25	48
Wild Cherry Dutch Ice	20 fl. oz.	330	0	0	0	0	35	69
Dutch Latté								
Caramel Dutch Latté	14 fl. oz.	350	15	11	0	55	170	49
Caramel Dutch Latté	20 fl. oz.	520	23	17	0	90	270	77
Coffee Dutch Latté	14 fl. oz.	290	14	9	0	50	135	38
Coffee Dutch Latté	20 fl. oz.	460	22	14	0	85	230	59
Mocha Dutch Latté	14 fl. oz.	360	17	11	0	55	135	47
Mocha Dutch Latté	20 fl. oz.	530	26	16	0	85	230	68
Dutch Shakes								
Chocolate Dutch Shake	14 fl. oz.	580	27	18	0	105	380	75
Chocolate Dutch Shake	20 fl. oz.	860	41	26	0	155	576	113
Coffee Dutch Shake	14 fl. oz.	590	27	18	0	105	304	77
Coffee Dutch Shake	20 fl. oz.	890	41	26	0	155	456	115
Strawberry Dutch Shake	14 fl. oz.	610	27	18	0	105	304	78
Strawberry Dutch Shake	20 fl. oz.	910	41	26	0	155	456	118
Vanilla Dutch Shake	14 fl. oz.	510	27	17	0	105	300	58
Vanilla Dutch Shake	20 fl. oz.	770	41	26	0	155	460	87
Dutch Smoothies								
Grape Dutch Smoothie	14 fl. oz.	230	82	5	0	30	100	36
Grape Dutch Smoothie	20 fl. oz.	400	14	9	0	55	180	65
Kiwi-Banana Dutch Smoothie	14 fl. oz.	240	8	5	0	30	100	38
Kiwi-Banana Dutch Smoothie	20 fl. oz.	430	14	9	0	55	180	68
Lemonade Dutch Smoothie	14 fl. oz.	300	8	5	0	30	80	53
Lemonade Dutch Smoothie	20 fl. oz.	540	14	9	0	55	150	95
Mocha Dutch Smoothie	14 fl. oz.	330	13	9	0	30	130	50
Mocha Dutch Smoothie	20 fl. oz.	590	23	16	0	55	240	90
Orange Crème Dutch Smoothie	14 fl. oz.	280	8	5	0	30	100	46
Orange Crème Dutch Smoothie	20 fl. oz.	500	14	9	0	55	180	83
Piña Colada Dutch Smoothie	14 fl. oz.	260	8	5	0	30	90	44
Piña Colada Dutch Smoothie	20 fl. oz.	470	14	9	0	55	170	79
Blue Raspberry Dutch Smoothie	14 fl. oz.	230	8	5	0	30	100	34
Blue Raspberry Dutch Smoothie	20 fl. oz.	400	14	9	0	55	180	61
Strawberry Dutch Smoothie	14 fl. oz.	250	8	5	0	30	100	40
Strawberry Dutch Smoothie	20 fl. oz.	450	14	9	0	55	180	72
Wild Cherry Dutch Smoothie	14 fl. oz.	250	8	5	0	30	90	41
Wild Cherry Dutch Smoothie	20 fl. oz.	450	14	9	0	55	170	74

Baja Fresh®

Fajita Burritos	Serving	Calories	Total fat (gm)	Saturated fat (gm)	Trans fats (gm)	Cholesterol (mg)	Sodium (mg)	Carbs (gm)
Charbroiled Mahi Mahi	1 item	890	38	16	1	120	1710	NA
Charbroiled Chicken	1 item	890	38	16	1	125	2010	NA
Charbroiled Steak	1 item	990	45	20	1.5	155	2020	NA
Savory Pork Carnitas	1 item	930	45	19	1	120	2150	NA
Charbroiled Shrimp	1 item	870	37	16	1	300	2100	NA
Breaded Fish	1 item	950	44	17	1.5	85	1770	NA
Bare Burrito (no tortilla)								
Charbroiled Chicken	1 item	640	7	1	0	75	2330	97
Charbroiled Steak	1 item	730	15	5	0.5	100	2350	99
Savory Pork Carnitas	1 item	680	14	4	0	70	2480	99
Veggie & Cheese	1 item	580	10	4	0	15	1990	101
Baja Burrito								
Charbroiled Chicken	1 item	930	45	16	1	120	2170	65
Charbroiled Steak	1 item	1030	52	19	2	145	2190	67
Savory Pork Carnitas	1 item	970	52	18	1.5	115	2320	67
Charbroiled Shrimp	1 item	910	44	16	1	295	2270	66
Breaded Fish	1 item	990	51	16	2	80	1940	78
Charbroiled Mahi Mahi	1 item	930	44	16	1	115	1870	66
Burrito Mexicano								
Charbroiled Chicken	1 item	940	20	4	0.5	75	2310	117
Charbroiled Steak	1 item	1030	27	8	1	100	2320	118
Savory Pork Carnitas	1 item	980	27	7	0.5	70	2450	119
Charbroiled Shrimp	1 item	920	20	4	0	245	2400	117
Breaded Fish	1 item	1000	26	5	1	30	2070	129
Charbroiled Mahi Mahi	1 item	930	20	4	0.5	70	2010	117
Burrito Ultimo								
Charbroiled Chicken	1 item	1030	43	19	1.5	135	2220	84
Charbroiled Steak	1 item	1120	50	22	2	165	2240	85
Savory Pork Carnitas	1 item	1070	50	21	1.5	130	2370	86
Charbroiled Shrimp	1 item	1010	43	19	1.5	310	2320	85
Breaded Fish	1 item	1090	49	19	2	95	1990	96
Charbroiled Mahi Mahi	1 item	1020	43	19	1.5	130	1920	84
Bean & Cheese								
No Meat	1 item	980	40	18	1.5	65	1820	96
Charbroiled Chicken	1 item	1120	42	18	1.5	140	2260	96
Charbroiled Steak	1 item	1210	49	22	2	165	2280	97
Savory Pork Carnitas	1 item	1160	49	21	1.5	130	2410	98
Breaded Fish	1 item	1180	48	19	2	95	2030	108

Baja Fresh®
Continued

Bean & Cheese continued	Serving	Calories	Total fat (gm)	Saturated fat (gm)	Trans fats (gm)	Cholesterol (mg)	Sodium (mg)	Carbs (gm)
Charbroiled Mahi Mahi	1 item	1110	41	18	1.5	130	1960	96
Charbroiled Shrimp	1 item	1090	41	18	1.5	310	2360	96
Grilled Veggie	1 item	950	40	18	1	65	1910	94
Burrito "Dos Manos"								
Charbroiled Chicken	1 item	835	29	13	1	78	2060	94
Charbroiled Steak	1 item	885	33	14	1	90	2065	95
Savory Pork Carnitas	1 item	855	33	14	1	73	2130	95
Charbroiled Shrimp	1 item	855	30	13	1	223	2240	95
Breaded Fish	1 item	965	37	13	1.25	70	2045	107
Charbroiled Mahi Mahi	1 item	855	30	13	1	85	1935	95
Tacos								
Charbroiled Chicken	1 item	250	8	1	0	25	240	28
Charbroiled Steak	1 item	280	10	2	0	30	240	28
Savory Pork Carnitas	1 item	260	11	2	0	20	290	29
Charbroiled Shrimp	1 item	250	8	1	0	90	290	28
Breaded Fish	1 item	320	16	2.5	0.5	15	400	27
Charbroiled Fish	1 item	300	12	2	0	20	280	26
Salads								
Charbroiled Chicken	1 item	590	22	6	1	105	1110	NA
Charbroiled Steak	1 item	700	31	11	2	135	1140	NA
Savory Pork Carnitas	1 item	640	30	10	1.5	95	1280	NA
Charbroiled Chicken Ensalada	1 item	310	7	2	0	110	1210	NA
Charbroiled Steak Ensalada	1 item	450	18	7	1	150	1240	NA
Savory Pork Carnitas Ensalada	1 item	370	18	6	0	100	1410	NA
Charbroiled Shrimp Ensalada	1 item	230	6	2	0	250	1110	NA
Side Salad	1 item	130	50	1.5	0	5	430	16
Soups								
w/o Charbroiled Chicken	1 item	270	14	4	0	15	2600	29
w/ Charbroiled Chicken	1 item	320	14	4	0	40	2750	29
"Side-by-Side"								
Charbroiled Chicken	1 item	500	27	8	0	150	1310	12
Charbroiled Steak	1 item	620	42	14	1	160	1550	14
Savory Pork Carnitas	1 item	570	40	13	0	140	1560	16
Tostadas								
No Meat	1 item	1010	53	13	1	40	1930	98
Charbroiled Chicken	1 item	1140	55	14	1	115	2370	98
Charbroiled Steak	1 item	1230	63	17	2	140	2380	98
Savory Pork Carnitas	1 item	1180	62	17	1	105	2520	100

Baja Fresh®
Continued

Tostadas continued

	Serving	Calories	Total fat (gm)	Saturated fat (gm)	Trans fats (gm)	Cholesterol (mg)	Sodium (mg)	Carbs (gm)
Charbroiled Shrimp	1 item	1120	55	14	1	285	2460	99
Breaded Fish	1 item	1200	61	15	1.5	70	2140	111
Charbroiled Fish	1 item	1130	55	14	1	105	2070	99
Fajitas								
Steak w/ flour tortillas	1 item	1430	50	16	1.5	170	3310	149
Steak w/ corn tortillas	1 item	1150	41	13	1.5	170	2470	107
Steak w/ mix tortillas	1 item	1360	47	15	1.5	170	3030	139
Chicken w/ flour tortillas	1 item	1290	40	11	0.5	130	3270	147
Chicken w/ corn tortillas	1 item	1010	31	8	0	130	2430	105
Chicken w/ mix tortillas	1 item	1210	37	10	0.5	130	3000	137
Carnitas w/ flour tortillas	1 item	1340	50	15	0.5	120	3480	150
Carnitas w/ corn tortillas	1 item	1070	41	12	0	120	2640	108
Carnitas w/ mix tortillas	1 item	1270	47	14	0.5	120	3200	140
Shrimp w/ flour tortillas	1 item	1260	39	11	0.5	390	3440	148
Shrimp w/ corn tortillas	1 item	990	30	8	0	390	2600	106
Shrimp w/ mix tortillas	1 item	1190	36	10	0.5	390	3170	138
Mahi Mahi w/ flour tortillas	1 item	1270	39	11	0.5	110	2830	147
Mahi Mahi w/ corn tortillas	1 item	990	30	8	0	110	1990	105
Mahi Mahi w/ mix tortillas	1 item	1200	36	10	0.5	110	2550	138
Breaded Fish w/ flour tortillas	1 item	1480	53	12	2	85	3050	172
Breaded Fish w/ corn tortillas	1 item	1210	44	10	1.5	85	2210	130
Breaded Fish w/ mix tortillas	1 item	1410	50	11	2	85	2770	162
Quesadilla								
Cheese	1 item	1200	78	37	2.5	140	2140	84
Veggie	1 item	1260	78	37	2.5	145	2310	96
Charbroiled Steak	1 item	1430	87	41	3	240	2600	84
Charbroiled Chicken	1 item	1330	80	37	2.5	215	2590	84
Savory Pork Carnitas	1 item	1370	87	40	2.5	205	2730	86
Charbroiled Shrimp	1 item	1310	79	37	2.5	385	2680	84
Breaded Fish	1 item	1400	86	38	3	170	2350	96
Charbroiled Mahi Mahi	1 item	1330	79	37	2.5	205	2290	84
Taquitos								
Chicken Taquitos w/ beans	1 item	780	40	12	1	85	1810	68
Chicken Taquitos w/ rice	1 item	740	40	11	1	85	1770	66
Steak Taquitos w/ beans	1 item	800	42	14	1	95	1760	NA
Steak Taquitos w/ rice	1 item	770	42	13	1	95	1720	NA
Nachos								
Cheese	1 item	1890	108	40	4	155	2530	163

Baja Fresh®
Continued

Nachos continued

	Serving	Calories	Total fat (gm)	Saturated fat (gm)	Trans fats (gm)	Cholesterol (mg)	Sodium (mg)	Carbs (gm)
Charbroiled Steak	1 item	2120	118	44	4.5	255	2990	163
Charbroiled Chicken	1 item	2020	110	41	4	230	2980	164
Savory Pork Carnitas	1 item	2060	117	43	4	220	3120	166
Charbroiled Shrimp	1 item	2000	110	41	4	395	3060	164
Breaded Fish	1 item	2090	116	41	4.5	185	2740	176
Charbroiled Mahi Mahi	1 item	2020	110	41	4	220	2680	164

Kid's Favorites

	Serving	Calories	Total fat (gm)	Saturated fat (gm)	Trans fats (gm)	Cholesterol (mg)	Sodium (mg)	Carbs (gm)
Kid's Chicken Taquitos	1 item	700	37	7	1	70	1000	60
Kid's Mini Bean & Cheese Burrito	1 item	620	18	7	0.5	25	1060	84
Kid's Mini Bean & Cheese Burrito w/ chicken	1 item	660	18	7	0.5	50	1220	84
Kid's Mini Cheese Quesadilla	1 item	610	26	13	1	50	940	72
Kid's Mini Cheese Quesadilla w/ chicken	1 item	650	27	13	1	75	1090	72

Side Orders

	Serving	Calories	Total fat (gm)	Saturated fat (gm)	Trans fats (gm)	Cholesterol (mg)	Sodium (mg)	Carbs (gm)
Chips & Guacamole	1 item	1340	83	8	2.5	0	950	141
Pronto Guacamole	1 item	560	34	3	1	0	370	60
Salsa Baja	8 oz.	70	2.5	0	0	0	970	7
Salsa Verde	8 oz.	50	0	0	0	0	1170	11
Salsa Roja	8 oz.	70	1	0	0	0	1080	13
Pico de Gallo	8 oz.	50	0.5	0	0	0	890	12
Chips & Salsa Baja	1 item	810	37	4	1.5	0	1140	98
Black Beans	1 item	360	2.5	1	0	5	1120	61
Pinto Beans	1 item	320	1	0	0	5	840	56
Rice	1 item	280	4	0.5	0	0	980	55
Rice & Beans Plate	1 item	420	5	1.5	0	10	1320	72
Side of Guacamole	3 oz.	110	13	1	0	0	270	5
Side of Guacamole	8 oz.	310	35	3	0	0	710	14
Veggie Mix	1 item	110	0	0	0	0	330	24
Charbroiled Steak	1 item	330	14	6	1	145	670	0
Charbroiled Chicken	1 item	230	3.5	0.5	0	125	760	0
Savory Pork Carnitas	1 item	300	16	6	0	110	1010	4
Charbroiled Shrimp	1 item	150	2	0.5	0	335	740	1
Breaded Fish	1 item	390	16	2.5	1.5	60	410	25
Charbroiled Fish	1 item	210	3	1	0	110	240	NA
Tostada Shell	1 item	490	28	3.5	0.5	0	600	44
Corn Tortilla Chips	1 oz.	150	7	0.5	0	0	35	29
Corn Tortilla Chips	5 oz.	740	34	3.5	1.5	0	170	90

Baskin-Robbins®

Ice Cream (regular scoop)

	Serving	Calories	Total fat (gm)	Saturated fat (gm)	Trans fats (gm)	Cholesterol (mg)	Sodium (mg)	Carbs (gm)
Butter Pecan	1 scoop	280	18	9	NA	50	95	NA
Chocolate	1 scoop	260	14	9	0	50	130	33
Chocolate Chip	1 scoop	270	16	10	0	55	95	28
Chocolate Chip Cookie Dough	1 scoop	290	15	9	1	55	130	36
Oreo Cookies 'n Cream	1 scoop	280	15	8	1	50	150	32
French Vanilla	1 scoop	280	18	11	1	120	85	26
Pralines 'n Cream	1 scoop	270	14	8	0	45	170	34
Rocky Road	1 scoop	290	15	8	0	45	120	36
Vanilla	1 scoop	260	16	10	1	65	70	26
Very Berry Strawberry	1 scoop	220	11	7	0	40	70	28
Espresso 'n Cream	1 scoop	180	4	2	0	10	120	NA
No Sugar Low-Fat Ice Cream								
Berries 'n Banana	1 scoop	110	2	1	0	10	125	NA
Pineapple Coconut	1 scoop	150	2	2	0	10	105	NA
Tin Roof Sundae	1 scoop	190	3	2	0	10	105	NA
Other Assorted Flavors	1 scoop	170	5	2	0	10	130	NA
Frozen Yogurt (assorted flavors)								
Low-Fat	1 scoop	190	4	2	0	10	150	35
Non-Fat	1 scoop	120	0	0	0	0	85	32
Truly Free	1 scoop	90	0	0	0	5	85	15
Ices								
Assorted Flavors	½ cup	130	0	0	0	0	15	33
Sherbert								
Assorted Flavors	1 scoop	160	2	2	0	10	40	34
Bold Breezes								
Strawberry Citrus Bold Breeze	16 fl. oz.	350	1	0	0	0	10	89
Wild Mango Bold Breeze	16 fl. oz.	340	1	0	0	0	10	84
Cappuccino Blasts								
Cappuccino Blast	16 fl. oz.	300	12	7	0	45	95	48
Cappuccino Blast/Low-Fat	16 fl. oz.	220	2	2	0	10	45	45

Bennigan's Irish American Grill & Tavern®
Does not provide nutrition information.

Blimpie®

	Serving	Calories	Total fat (gm)	Saturated fat (gm)	Trans fats (gm)	Cholesterol (mg)	Sodium (mg)	Carbs (gm)
6" Hot Sub								
Grilled Chicken	1 item	370	9	3	0	35	840	NA
GrilleMax	1 item	410	6	2	0	5	830	NA
Meatball	1 item	570	27	9	0	60	1140	NA
MexiMax	1 item	430	9	2	0	0	1010	NA
Pastrami	1 item	510	17	7	0	75	1660	NA
Pastrami Special	1 item	460	14	6	0	45	1440	NA
Steak & Onion Melt	1 item	440	16	6	0	70	1060	NA
VegiMax	1 item	390	7	2	0	0	980	NA
6" Cold Sub								
Blimpie Best	1 item	440	15	6	0	55	1450	NA
Buffalo Chicken	1 item	400	8	3	0	60	2110	NA
Club	1 item	410	11	5	0	55	1210	NA
Ham & Swiss Cheese	1 item	410	12	5	0	50	1150	NA
Roast Beef	1 item	450	13	6	0	60	1270	NA
Seafood	1 item	350	8	2	0	20	900	NA
BLT	1 item	590	32	10	0	40	1600	NA
Tuna	1 item	490	23	4	0	50	880	NA
Turkey	1 item	420	11	5	0	60	1600	NA
6" Panini Grilled Sub								
Beef, Turkey, & Cheddar	1 item	600	31	10	0	70	1840	NA
Corned Beef Reuben	1 item	630	33	5	0	45	1910	NA
Cuban	1 item	460	12	6	0	65	1530	NA
Turkey Italiano	1 item	390	10	4	0	50	1800	NA
Ultimate Club	1 item	720	42	13	0	80	1930	NA
Wraps								
Beef & Cheddar	1 wrap	710	37	11	0	80	2180	NA
Chicken Caesar	1 wrap	650	35	7	0	45	1640	NA
Southwestern	1 wrap	670	35	8	0	55	2500	NA
Steak & Onion	1 wrap	720	37	10	0	80	1720	NA
Ultimate BLT	1 wrap	830	50	15	0	80	2680	NA
Zesty Italian	1 wrap	680	33	10	0	60	2370	NA
Breads (6" roll)								
Italian White Roll	1 roll	240	4	1	0	0	480	NA
Poppy White	1 roll	250	4	1	0	0	480	NA
Sesame White	1 roll	250	5	1	0	0	480	NA
Wheat	1 roll	230	4	1	0	0	460	NA
Poppy Wheat	1 roll	240	4	>1	0	0	460	NA
Sesame Wheat	1 roll	250	5	1	0	0	460	NA

Blimpie® Continued

Breads (6" roll) continued

	Serving	Calories	Total fat (gm)	Saturated fat (gm)	Trans fats (gm)	Cholesterol (mg)	Sodium (mg)	Carbs (gm)
Honey Oat	1 roll	300	7	1	0	0	460	NA
Marble Rye	1 roll	300	3	1	0	0	700	NA
Zesty Parmesan	1 roll	270	5	2	0	5	550	NA
Flat Bread	1 roll	270	9	2	0	0	290	NA
Traditional Wrap	1 wrap	320	8	2	0	0	820	NA
Spinach & Herb Wrap	1 wrap	310	8	2	0	0	780	NA
Salads (w/o dressing unless noted)								
Antipasto Salad	1 salad	240	13	6	NA	70	1220	NA
Chef Salad	1 salad	210	9	5	NA	65	960	NA
Chili Ole	1 salad	480	27	11	NA	45	1240	NA
Grilled Chicken w/ caesar dressing	1 salad	350	27	5	NA	45	860	NA
Roast Beef 'n Bleu	1 salad	390	16	10	NA	70	1550	NA
Seafood Salad	1 salad	120	5	1	NA	20	420	NA
Tuna Salad	1 salad	260	19	3	NA	50	400	NA
Zesto Pesto Turkey	1 salad	370	19	8	NA	40	1410	NA
Soups								
Grande Chili w/ beans & beef	8 oz.	250	7	4	NA	40	1230	NA
Chicken Noodle	8 oz.	120	3	1	NA	20	850	NA
Chicken & Rice	8 oz.	230	12	2	NA	30	1210	NA
Cream of Broccoli & Cheese	8 oz.	190	12	5	NA	15	940	NA
Cream of Potato	8 oz.	190	9	3	NA	0	860	NA
Garden Vegetable	8 oz.	80	1	0	NA	0	620	NA
Vegetable Beef	8 oz.	80	2	1	NA	5	1010	NA
Side Items								
Cole Slaw	5 oz.	180	13	2	NA	5	230	NA
Macaroni Salad	5 oz.	360	25	4	NA	10	660	NA
Mustard Potato Salad	5 oz.	160	5	1	NA	5	660	NA
Potato Salad	5 oz.	270	19	3	NA	10	560	NA

Fast Food Factoid:

Nobody's hiding anything at Baskin-Robbins. It's yummy, delicious, full-flavor ice cream, and all the ice cream is coded red because it should be eaten sparingly.

Bob Evans®

Breakfast Combinations

	Serving	Calories	Total fat (gm)	Saturated fat (gm)	Trans fats (gm)	Cholesterol (mg)	Sodium (mg)	Carbs (gm)
Border Scramble Burritto	1 meal	1100	64	21	1	561	1999	80
Lite Sausage Breakfast	1 meal	469	21	5	0	20	420	NA
Country Biscuit w/ sausage	1 meal	852	49	16	NA	261	2455	NA
Country Biscuit Breakfast	1 meal	659	45	16	6	270	1700	40
Country Fried Steak	1 meal	481	33	12	0	60	1215	NA
Fruit & Yogurt Plate	1 meal	414	2	1	0	5	106	93
Pot Roast Hash Breakfast	1 meal	752	46	17	1	529	1261	34
Egg Beaters Omelette Shell	1 meal	173	12	2	0	5	581	3
Eggs Benedict w/ Canadian bacon	1 meal	418	20	5	1	442	1008	NA
Bacon & Cheese Omelette	1 meal	825	66	25	0	826	1603	6
Cheese Omelette	1 meal	477	40	15	1	530	428	4
Ham & Cheese Omelette	1 meal	505	39	13	1	546	1278	3
Sausage & Cheese Omelette	1 meal	679	57	20	1	554	1030	3
Sausage Country Benedict	1 meal	936	66	24	5	536	2098	40
Southwestern Chicken Omelette	1 meal	674	51	17	1	590	1669	3
Spinach, Bacon, & Tomato Country Benedict	1 meal	729	48	16	5	494	1885	42
Sunshine Skillet	1 meal	842	60	18	3	819	1474	36
Western Omelette	1 meal	522	39	13	1	546	1279	8

Breakfast Meats

	Serving	Calories	Total fat (gm)	Saturated fat (gm)	Trans fats (gm)	Cholesterol (mg)	Sodium (mg)	Carbs (gm)
Bacon	1 strip	36	4	2	0	5	54	NA
Canadian Bacon	1 slice	21	1	0	0	9	261	NA
Smoked Ham	1 slice	66	2	1	0	40	857	2
Sausage Link	1 link	125	11	3	0	14	184	0
Lite Sausage Link	1 link	100	7	19	0	19	278	0
Sausage Patty	1 patty	117	9	4	0	22	279	0

Waffles & Pancakes (w/o syrup or toppings)

	Serving	Calories	Total fat (gm)	Saturated fat (gm)	Trans fats (gm)	Cholesterol (mg)	Sodium (mg)	Carbs (gm)
Belgium Waffle	1 item	342	10	4	3	18	735	NA
Buttermilk Hotcake	1 item	171	5	2	2	9	367	53
Blueberry Hotcake	1 item	187	5	2	2	9	369	55
Stuffed Hotcakes	1 item	1500	70	28	9	55	2200	198
Multigrain Hotcake	1 item	322	10	3	1	0	773	52
French Toast	1 item	131	2	0	0	25	175	13

Breakfast Side Items

	Serving	Calories	Total fat (gm)	Saturated fat (gm)	Trans fats (gm)	Cholesterol (mg)	Sodium (mg)	Carbs (gm)
English Muffin	1 item	139	1	0	0	0	229	NA
Wheat or White Toast w/ butter	1 slice	115	7	1	0	0	188	NA
Texas Toast	1 slice	120	1	0	0	0	125	NA
Biscuit (plain)	1 item	277	12	3	2	0	764	NA
Sausage Gravy	7 oz.	217	15	9	0	18	901	21

Bob Evans®
Continued

Breakfast Side Items continued

	Serving	Calories	Total fat (gm)	Saturated fat (gm)	Trans fats (gm)	Cholesterol (mg)	Sodium (mg)	Carbs (gm)
Scrambled Eggs	2 eggs	170	11	3	0	482	142	3
EggBeaters	4.5 oz.	149	12	2	0	3	423	3
Fruit Cup	9.25 oz	164	1	0	0	0	11	38
Home Fries	5 oz.	193	7	1	1	0	577	27
Oatmeal (plain)	12 oz.	185	3	0	0	0	301	32
Entrée Items								
Hamburger	1 item	605	38	25	2	82	429	31
Cheeseburger	1 item	707	47	21	2	112	905	32
Bacon Cheeseburger	1 item	778	54	24	2	122	1014	32
Bob's BLT	1 item	751	51	19	1	279	1266	27
Chicken Salad Sandwich	1 item	643	38	6	0	62	1273	53
Double Sausage Sandwich	1 item	717	46	18	0	91	1743	31
Fried Chicken item	1 item	508	23	4	1	77	1032	43
Grilled Cheese Sandwich	1 item	396	16	6	1	29	777	25
Grilled Chicken Sandwich	1 item	442	17	3	1	90	947	30
Fish Market Haddock Sandwich	1 item	520	19	3	2	32	889	78
Meatloaf Sandwich	1 item	716	38	17	1	144	3403	NA
Pot Roast item	1 item	655	31	12	0	98	1455	58
Pulled Pork Sandwich	1 item	464	18	2	0	59	579	NA
Slow Roasted Pork Loin Sandwich	1 item	844	48	19	1	140	2491	58
Slow Roasted Turkey Bacon Melt	1 item	617	29	11	1	87	1818	53
Slow Roasted Turkey	1 item	696	36	12	1	80	2439	NA
Steak Burger	1 item	539	32	11	22	96	756	NA
Lunch Savors Meals								
Steak Tips & Noodles	15 oz.	581	26	6	1	135	1802	23
Grilled Chicken Stir-Fry	16 oz.	497	18	4	NA	66	1295	44
Vegetable Stir-Fry	13 oz.	278	4	1	NA	0	855	44
Lunch Savors Salads (w/o dressing or toppings)								
Cobb Salad w/ grilled chicken	1 salad	547	39	16	0	319	1321	10
Country Spinach Salad w/ grilled chicken	1 salad	545	38	10	0	282	1106	11
Frisco Salad w/ grilled chicken	1 salad	461	31	12	0	115	1040	NA
Wildfire Chicken Salad w/ fried chicken	1 salad	646	29	9	0	52	1184	81
Kid's Meals								
Lil' Farmer's Breakfast	1 meal	446	26	8	NA	261	774	NA
Plenty-O Pancakes	1 order	503	17	9	4	24	982	NA
Hot Diggety Dog	1 item	361	26	10	NA	39	843	NA
Mini Cheeseburger	1 item	252	14	4	0	25	288	NA
Pizza Pizzazz	1 order	505	23	8	NA	18	796	NA

Bob Evans®
Continued
Kid's Meals continued

	Serving	Calories	Total fat (gm)	Saturated fat (gm)	Trans fats (gm)	Cholesterol (mg)	Sodium (mg)	Carbs (gm)
Mac & Cheese	6 .5 oz.	330	12	4	2	20	610	45
Chicken Quesadilla	1 item	547	31	12	NA	73	1160	NA
Spaghetti & Meatballs	10.5 oz.	523	21	9	NA	51	999	NA
Smiley Face Potatoes	6 oz.	340	13	1	1	0	780	57
Senior Meals (entrée Only)								
Spaghetti & Meatballs	11.5 oz.	617	29	11	NA	69	1166	NA
Grilled Chicken Stir-Fry	16 oz.	480	18	4	4	57	1236	44
Steak Tips & Noodles	14.5 oz	573	26	6	1	135	1733	23
Farm Fresh Salads (w/o dressing or toppings)								
Garden Side Salad	1 salad	152	4	0	0	0	396	22
Chicken Salad Plate	1 salad	781	46	7	0	87	1132	72
Chili & Cheese Taco Salad	1 salad	928	62	18	0	91	1724	NA
Cobb Salad w/ grilled chicken	1 salad	753	50	20	0	360	1708	14
Country Spinach Salad w/ grilled chicken	1 salad	624	40	10	0	314	1350	13
Cranberry Pecan Chicken Salad	1 salad	1140	64	20	0	123	3007	63
Fresh Garden Salad	1 salad	137	4	0	0	0	347	22
Frisco Salad w/ grilled chicken	1 salad	595	38	13	NA	148	1272	NA
Frisco Salad w/ fried chicken	1 salad	648	38	12	NA	91	1577	NA
Fruit & Yogurt Plate	1 salad	398	2	1	0	5	109	92
Heritage Chef Salad	1 salad	456	26	12	0	286	1582	14
Wildfire Chicken Salad w/ grilled chicken	1 salad	745	36	10	0	122	1213	53
Wildfire Chicken Salad w/ fried chicken	1 salad	798	36	10	0	66	1518	77
Beef & Pork Dinners (entrée only)								
Country Fried Steak w/o gravy	5.25 oz.	481	33	12	0	60	1217	31
Meatloaf	9.5 oz.	630	44	19	1	157	1081	9
Open-Faced Roast Beef Dinner	9 oz.	453	25	9	0	104	1042	24
Pork Chop Dinner (plain)	6.25 oz.	477	28	9	NA	129	829	NA
Steak Monterey	9 oz.	600	41	17	0	126	1671	NA
Steak Tips & Noodles	27.5 oz.	1027	39	10	1	268	3230	44
Chicken & Turkey Dinners (entrée only)								
Chicken-n-Noodles	14.5 oz.	407	22	5	0	15	659	67
Chicken Pot Pie	1 item	758	49	22	12	209	1754	64
Chicken Parmesan	22.9 oz	651	33	10	0	127	3012	45
Chicken Stir-Fry	26 oz	636	20	4	0	75	2681	77
Fried Chicken Dinner	5 oz.	291	15	3	0	77	666	13
Grilled Chicken Dinner (plain)	4.5 oz.	214	9	2	1	84	544	0
Steak Tips Stir-Fry	30 oz	1020	47	11	0	170	3641	84

	Serving	Calories	Total fat (gm)	Saturated fat (gm)	Trans fats (gm)	Cholesterol (mg)	Sodium (mg)	Carbs (gm)
Chicken & Turkey Dinners (entrée only) continued								
Turkey & Dressing	14.5 oz.	549	25	7	13	126	1407	33
Wildfire Grilled Chicken Breast	5.7 oz	325	13	3	0	85	784	NA
Pasta & Stir-Fry Dinners (entrée only)								
Buttered Pasta Noodles	5.5 oz.	287	13	2	NA	47	120	NA
Italian Sausage & Pepper Pasta	22 oz	636	40	12	0	64	3040	NA
Spaghetti w/ marinara sauce	16.5 oz.	619	7	3	NA	15	1128	NA
Spaghetti & Meatballs	21 oz.	1087	45	17	NA	107	1965	NA
Stir-Fried Grilled Chicken	23.5 oz.	727	27	5	NA	85	1962	77
Stir-Fried Vegetables	26 oz.	502	7	1	NA	5	1416	86
Seafood Dinners (entrée only)								
Atlantic Salmon Fillet Dinner	29 oz	800	35	10	0	125	2200	NA
Grilled Catfish, New Orleans-Style	4.5 oz.	270	19	3	NA	58	896	NA
Grilled Shrimp Dinner	28 oz	700	35	10	0	300	2800	NA
Lemon Pepper Cod	4 oz.	271	16	3	NA	56	598	NA
Potato-Crusted Flounder	4 1/2 oz	254	17	4	0	25	552	8
Salmon w/ garlic herb butter	6.5 oz.	424	28	5	1	75	467	2
Dinner Side Items								
Dinner Roll	1 roll	201	5	1	0	9	268	NA
Garlic Bread	1 item	218	16	3	NA	0	386	NA
Broccoli Florets	5.5 oz.	44	1	0	0	0	41	6
Glazed Carrots	4.5 oz	137	6	2	3	7	125	14
Buttered Corn	4.5 oz.	156	9	3	NA	12	313	25
Coleslaw	4 oz.	198	13	2	0	12	229	19
French Fries	5 oz.	217	7	2	2	0	300	51
Green Beans w/ ham	4.5 oz.	53	2	1	0	7	641	NA
Baked Potato (plain)	1 item	207	0	0	0	0	16	54
Mashed Potatoes	5 oz.	121	6	4	0	18	382	17
Beef Gravy	3 oz.	33	2	0	0	2	560	3
Chicken Gravy	3 oz.	71	6	2	0	4	460	3
Country Gravy	3 oz.	54	4	1	4	0	546	6
Onion Rings	6 oz.	461	27	5	NA	1	680	NA
Rice Pilaf	5 oz	163	3	1	NA	0	606	20
Grilled Veggies	10 oz.	283	20	4	0	0	203	14

Fast Food Factoid:
If all smokers in the United States today quit smoking, there would be a 30% reduction in all cancers.

Bojangles®

Cajun Spice Chicken

	Serving	Calories	Total fat (gm)	Saturated fat (gm)	Trans fats (gm)	Cholesterol (mg)	Sodium (mg)	Carbs (gm)
Breast	1 item	278	17	NA	NA	75	565	12
Leg	1 item	264	16	NA	NA	96	530	11
Thigh	1 item	310	23	NA	NA	67	465	11
Wing	1 item	355	25	NA	NA	94	630	11

Southern Style Chicken

	Serving	Calories	Total fat (gm)	Saturated fat (gm)	Trans fats (gm)	Cholesterol (mg)	Sodium (mg)	Carbs (gm)
Breast	1 item	261	16	NA	NA	76	702	12
Leg	1 item	254	15	NA	NA	94	446	11
Thigh	1 item	308	21	NA	NA	78	630	14
Wing	1 item	337	21	NA	NA	86	684	19

Biscuit Items

	Serving	Calories	Total fat (gm)	Saturated fat (gm)	Trans fats (gm)	Cholesterol (mg)	Sodium (mg)	Carbs (gm)
Bacon	1 item	290	17	5	NA	10	810	26
Bacon, Egg & Cheese	1 item	550	42	14	NA	160	1250	27
Cajun Fillet	1 item	454	21	6	NA	41	949	46
Country Ham	1 item	270	15	4	NA	20	1010	26
Egg	1 item	400	30	6	NA	120	630	26
Sausage	1 item	350	23	7	NA	20	810	26
Smoked Sausage	1 item	380	26	9	NA	20	940	27
Steak	1 item	649	49	13	NA	34	1126	37

Items

	Serving	Calories	Total fat (gm)	Saturated fat (gm)	Trans fats (gm)	Cholesterol (mg)	Sodium (mg)	Carbs (gm)
Cajun Fillet item	1 item	337	11	5	NA	45	401	41
Grilled Fillet item	1 item	235	5	3	NA	51	540	25

Individual Fixins'

	Serving	Calories	Total fat (gm)	Saturated fat (gm)	Trans fats (gm)	Cholesterol (mg)	Sodium (mg)	Carbs (gm)
Biscuit (plain)	1 item	243	12	3	NA	2	663	29
Bo-berry Sweet Biscuits	1 order	220	10	3	NA	<1	410	29
Botato Rounds	1 order	235	11	4	NA	13	328	31
Buffalo Bites	1 order	180	5	2	NA	105	720	5
Cajun Pintos	1 order	110	0	0	NA	0	480	NA
Chicken Supremes	1 order	340	16	6	NA	58	630	26
Cinnamon Sweet Biscuits	1 order	320	1	4	NA	<1	560	37
Marinated Cole Slaw	1 order	136	3	0	NA	0	454	26
Corn on the Cob	1 item	140	2	0	NA	0	20	34
Dirty Rice	1 order	166	6	2	NA	10	762	24
Green Beans	1 order	25	0	0	NA	0	710	5
Macaroni & Cheese	1 order	198	14	5	NA	26	418	12
Potatoes w/o gravy	1 order	80	1	0	NA	0	380	16
Seasoned Fries	1 order	344	19	5	NA	13	480	39

Boston Market®

	Serving	Calories	Total fat (gm)	Saturated fat (gm)	Trans fats (gm)	Cholesterol (mg)	Sodium (mg)	Carbs (gm)
Make Your Meal								
¼ White Original Rotisserie Chicken	9.3 oz.	510	27	9	0	255	1140	4
¼ White Original Rotisserie Chicken w/o skin	9.3 oz.	320	7	2	0	140	950	6
¼ White Simply Seasoned Chicken	9.2 oz.	510	27	9	0	255	1110	NA
¼ Dark Original Rotisserie Chicken	7 oz.	420	26	8	0	250	660	NA
¼ Dark Original Rotisserie Chicken w/o skin	7 oz.	400	21	6	0	240	700	NA
¼ Dark Simply Seasoned Chicken	7 oz.	420	26	8	0	250	630	NA
Roasted Turkey	5 oz.	230	10	1.5	0	45	620	NA
Pastry Top Chicken Pot Pie	15 oz.	800	49	18	0	125	910	60
USDA Choice All Beef Meatloaf	7.7 oz.	510	35	14	0	135	115	23
"Award Winning" Roasted Sirloin	5 oz.	270	10	3.5	7	125	290	0
Family Meals								
Spiral Sliced Holiday Ham	8 oz	450	26	10	0	70	620	NA
Whole Original Rotisserie Chicken	3 oz.	160	7	2	0	95	310	4
Whole Simply Seasoned Rotisserie Chicken	3 oz.	160	7	2	0	95	300	NA
Whole Holiday Turkey	6.7 oz.	310	18	5	0	135	940	0
Roasted Turkey	5 oz.	230	10	1.5	0	45	620	0
USDA Choice Beef Meatloaf	7.7 oz.	510	35	14	0	135	115	23
"Award Winning" Roasted Sirloin	5 oz.	270	10	3.5	1	125	290	0
Soups & Sides								
Sweet Corn	6.2 oz.	170	4	1	0	0	95	37
Creamed Spinach	6.7 oz.	280	23	15	0	70	580	12
Green Beans	4.7 oz.	90	5	1	0	0	70	7
Cinnamon Apples	5.1 oz.	210	3	0	0	0	15	47
Macaroni & Cheese	7.8 oz.	320	12	8	0	30	950	39
Mashed Potatoes	7.8 oz.	210	9	6	0	25	660	36
Poultry Gravy	2 oz.	25	1	0	0	0	350	4
Garlic Dill New Potatoes	5.5 oz.	140	3	1	0	0	120	4
Fresh Vegetable Stuffing	4.8 oz.	190	8	1	0	0	580	25
Sweet Potato Casserole	7 oz.	460	17	6	0	20	210	77
Fresh Steamed Vegetables	4.8 oz.	50	2	0	0	0	45	8
Garden Fresh Coleslaw	4.4 oz.	220	19	3	0	20	160	21
Seasonal Fresh Fruit Salad	5 oz.	60	0	0	0	0	20	15
Spincah Artichoke Dip	2 oz.	100	8	4	0	15	220	3
Caesar Side Salad	2.5 oz.	40	2	2	0	0	70	7

Boston Market®
Continued

Soups & Sides continued

	Serving	Calories	Total fat (gm)	Saturated fat (gm)	Trans fats (gm)	Cholesterol (mg)	Sodium (mg)	Carbs (gm)
Chicken Tortilla Soup	6 oz.	350	21	7	0	50	1040	24
Chicken Noodle Soup	6 oz.	180	7	2	0	60	200	17
Sandwiches								
Boston Sirloin Dip Carver	13 oz.	970	45	12	8	195	1510	70
Boston Chicken Carver	11 oz.	700	29	7	0	90	1560	68
Meatloaf Carver	15 oz.	960	45	18	0	155	1280	96
Boston Turkey Carver	13.7 oz.	830	36	8	0	90	1810	68
Boston Turkey Dip Carver	16 oz.	830	36	8	0	90	2470	67
Salads								
Caesar Salad Entrée	7.2 oz.	140	8	5	0	15	280	8
Caesar Salad Dressing	2.5 oz.	360	38	6	0.5	30	910	4
Market Chopped Salad w/o dressing	1 Salad	210	9	4	0	10	280	10
Market Chopped Salad dressing	2.5 oz.	360	39	6	1	0	1710	2
Market Chopped Salad w/ Rotisserie Chicken	3 oz.	310	11.5	4.5	0	55	580	13
Market Chopped Salad w/ Roasted Turkey	3 oz.	350	15	5	0	35	650	11
Market Chopped Salad w/ Roasted Sirloin	3 oz.	370	15	6	4	85	450	10
Desserts								
Apple Pie	1 slice	420	20	4	5	0	650	56
Chocolate Cake	1 slice	600	32	7	5	65	210	75
Chocolate Chip Fudge Brownie	1 brownie	580	23	5	0	90	390	81
Cornbread	2 oz.	180	5	2	2	10	320	31
Nestle Tollhouse Chocolate Chip Cookie	1 cookie	370	19	8	0	20	340	49

Buffalo Wild Wings Grill & Bar®
Does not provide nutrition information.

NOTES:

_____

_____

_____

_____

_____

_____

_____

Burger King®

	Serving	Calories	Total fat (gm)	Saturated fat (gm)	Trans fats (gm)	Cholesterol (mg)	Sodium (mg)	Carbs (gm)
Breakfast								
Bacon, Egg, & Cheese Biscuit	1 item	410	25	8	5	150	1320	31
Cini-minis	1 item	390	18	5	4	20	560	51
Croissan'wich w/ egg & cheese	1 item	300	17	6	2	195	700	26
Croissan'wich w/ bacon, egg & cheese	1 item	340	18	6	2	210	1470	26
Croissan'wich w/ sausage, egg & cheese	1 item	500	36	12	2	220	1060	26
Croissan'wich w/ sausage & cheese	1 item	410	29	11	2	45	830	26
Double Croissan'wich w/ bacon, egg & cheese	1 item	430	26	11	2	220	1360	27
Double Croissan'wich w/ ham, egg & cheese	1 item	420	23	9	2	235	2450	27
Double Croissan'wich w/ sausage, egg & cheese	1 item	750	60	21	3	260	1630	26
Double Croissan'wich w/ ham, bacon, egg & cheese	1 item	420	25	10	2	225	1910	27
Double Croissan'wich w/ ham, sausage, egg & cheese	1 item	580	41	15	3	245	2040	27
Double Croissan'wich w/ sausage, bacon, egg & cheese	1 item	590	43	16	3	240	1490	27
Enormous Omelette Sandwich	1 item	730	47	17	1	415	1860	44
French Toast Sticks	5 pieces	390	20	5	5	0	440	26
Ham, Egg, & Cheese Biscuit	1 item	390	22	7	5	145	1410	31
Ham Omelette Sandwich	1 item	330	14	5	0	90	1130	35
Hash Brown Rounds (small)	2.5 oz.	230	15	4	5	0	450	25
Sausage Biscuit	1 item	390	26	8	5	35	1020	28
Sausage, Egg, & Cheese Biscuit	1 item	530	37	12	6	175	1490	31
Burgers								
BK Double Stacker	1 item	610	39	16	2	125	1100	32
BK Triple Stacker	1 item	800	54	23	2	185	1450	33
BK Quad Stacker	1 item	1000	68	30	3	240	1800	34
Whopper	1 item	700	42	13	1	85	1020	51
Whopper w/ cheese	1 item	800	49	18	2	110	1450	51
Double Whopper	1 item	970	61	22	2	160	1110	52
Double Whopper w/ cheese	1 item	1060	69	27	3	185	1540	52
Triple Whopper	1 item	1130	74	27	3	255	1160	51
Triple Whopper w/ cheese	1 item	1230	82	32	3.5	275	1590	52
Whopper Jr.	1 item	390	22	7	1	45	550	31
Whopper Jr. w/ cheese	1 item	430	26	9	1	55	770	31
Hamburger	1 item	310	13	5	1	40	550	30
Cheeseburger	1 item	350	17	8	1	50	770	31
Double Hamburger	1 item	440	23	10	1	75	600	30

Burger King®
Continued
Burgers continued

	Serving	Calories	Total fat (gm)	Saturated fat (gm)	Trans fats (gm)	Cholesterol (mg)	Sodium (mg)	Carbs (gm)
Double Cheeseburger	1 item	530	31	15	2	100	1030	31
Bacon Cheeseburger	1 item	390	20	9	1	60	990	NA
Bacon Double Cheeseburger	1 item	570	34	17	2	110	1250	NA
BK Veggie Burger	1 item	380	16	3	0	5	930	46
Angus Steak Burger	1 item	570	22	8	1	180	1270	55
Angus Bacon & Cheese	1 item	710	33	15	2	215	1990	NA

Other Items

	Serving	Calories	Total fat (gm)	Saturated fat (gm)	Trans fats (gm)	Cholesterol (mg)	Sodium (mg)	Carbs (gm)
BK Fish Fillet	1 item	520	30	8	0	55	840	67
Chicken Whopper	1 item	570	25	5	0	75	1410	NA
Original Chicken item	1 item	560	28	6	2	60	1270	52
TenderCrisp Chicken Sandwich	1 item	780	45	7	4	55	1730	68
Spicy TenderCrisp Chicken Sandwich	1 item	720	37	6	4	50	1990	68

Salads & Side Items (w/o dressing)

	Serving	Calories	Total fat (gm)	Saturated fat (gm)	Trans fats (gm)	Cholesterol (mg)	Sodium (mg)	Carbs (gm)
Fire-Grilled Chicken Caesar Salad	1 salad	190	7	3	0	50	900	NA
Fire-Grilled Shrimp Caesar Salad	1 salad	180	10	3	1	120	880	NA
TenderCrisp Caesar Salad	1 salad	390	22	5	4	40	1160	NA
Fire-Grilled Chicken Garden Salad	1 salad	210	7	3	0	50	910	NA
Fire-Grilled Shrimp Garden Salad	1 salad	200	10	3	1	120	900	NA
TenderCrisp Garden Salad	1 salad	410	22	5	4	40	1170	26
Side Salad	1 salad	20	0	0	0	0	15	3
Motts Strawberry Flavor Applesauce	4 oz.	90	0	0	0	0	0	NA
Chicken Tenders	5 pieces	210	12	4	3	30	530	13
French Fries (medium)	4 oz.	360	18	5	5	0	640	41
Onion Rings (medium)	3.25 oz.	320	16	4	4	0	460	37
BK Chicken Fries	9 pieces	390	23	5	5	50	980	26
Cheesy Tots	9 pieces	320	18	7	3	30	970	NA

California Pizza Kitchen®
Pizza

	Serving	Calories	Total fat (gm)	Saturated fat (gm)	Trans fats (gm)	Cholesterol (mg)	Sodium (mg)	Carbs (gm)
Crispy Thin Crust Margherita	1/3 pizza	300	13	5	1	20	490	NA
Crispy Thin Crust Sicilian Recipe	1/3 pizza	310	14	5	0	30	890	NA
Crispy Thin Crust White	1/3 pizza	290	12	6	1	25	570	NA

Note: This was the only information provided.

Captain D's®

	Serving	Calories	Total fat (gm)	Saturated fat (gm)	Trans fats (gm)	Cholesterol (mg)	Sodium (mg)	Carbs (gm)
Broiled & Baked Entrées								
Chicken Breast	1 item	112	2	1	NA	62	741	NA
Fish	1 item	50	1	0	NA	3	204	NA
Salmon	1 item	326	12	0	NA	32	1200	NA
Shrimp	1 item	52	2	0	NA	68	148	NA
Fried Entrées								
Breaded Chicken Strip	1 item	114	6	2	NA	23	279	11
Stuffed Crab	1 item	1124	7	2	NA	16	220	9
Batter Dipped Fish	1 item	221	12	5	NA	34	520	10
Country Style Fish	1 item	84	4	1	NA	12	176	NA
Breaded Butterfly Shrimp	1 item	172	8	4	NA	44	484	3
Fried Pickles	1 item	360	30	NA	1	30	1810	17
Items								
Broiled/Baked Chicken w/o Creole Sauce	1 item	305	5	1	NA	61	1156	45
Fried Chicken w/ Creole sauce	1 item	617	22	8	NA	70	1363	67
Broiled/Baked Fish w/o tartar sauce	1 item	425	8	1	NA	10	1144	NA
Giant Fish Sandwich w/o tarter sauce	1 item	715	29	12	NA	69	1572	62
Captain's Catch w/o tarter sauce	1 item	477	21	9	NA	52	1224	NA
Salads (w/o dressing)								
Side Salad	1 salad	23	1	1	NA	0	14	NA
Garden Salad	1 salad	57	1	1	NA	6	98	9
Blackened Chicken Caesar Salad	1 salad	293	8	2	NA	127	1174	10
Fried Chicken Club Salad	1 salad	627	35	13	NA	105	1549	51
Oriental Broiled/Baked Shrimp Salad	1 salad	308	7	1	NA	175	442	NA
Oriental Fried Shrimp Salad	1 salad	550	23	7	NA	91	912	NA
Side Items								
Breadstick	1 item	150	6	2	NA	5	150	21
Steamed Broccoli	3 oz.	25	1	0	NA	0	25	5
Cheesesticks	1 order	457	25	11	NA	42	1066	32
Coleslaw	4 oz.	170	12	2	NA	10	305	13
Corn on the Cob	1 item	150	3	0	NA	0	20	37
French Fries (small)	3.5 oz.	298	14	5	NA	0	450	38
Garlic Mashed Potatoes	1 item	100	30	NA	0	<5	490	16
Gumbo Soup with Rice	1 item	210	8	NA	0	25	700	26
Seasoned Green Beans	4 oz.	90	3	1	NA	5	505	10
Hushpuppy	1 item	88	4	1	NA	10	244	36
Jalapeño Poppers	1 order	385	24	12	NA	47	1320	NA
Baked Potato (plain)	1 item	190	0	0	NA	0	15	54

Captain D's®
Continued
Side Items continued

	Serving	Calories	Total fat (gm)	Saturated fat (gm)	Trans fats (gm)	Cholesterol (mg)	Sodium (mg)	Carbs (gm)
Fried Okra	4 oz.	285	15	5	NA	15	551	23
Rice	4 oz.	180	1	0	NA	0	105	NA
Seasonal Vegetables	3.5 oz.	35	0	0	NA	0	15	9
Desserts								
Carrot Cake	1 item	370	15	3	NA	30	310	50
Chocolate Cake	1 item	310	12	3	NA	24	262	49
Pineapple Cream Cheese Pie	1 item	320	15	6	NA	15	310	43
Pecan Pie	1 item	490	22	4	NA	70	560	56

Fast Food Factoid:

It is useless for the sheep to pass resolutions in favor of vegetarianism while the wolf remains of a different opinion.

William Ralph Inge (1860–1954)

Carl's Jr.®
Breakfast

	Serving	Calories	Total fat (gm)	Saturated fat (gm)	Trans fats (gm)	Cholesterol (mg)	Sodium (mg)	Carbs (gm)
Sourdough Breakfast Sandwich	1 item	410	19	9	NA	255	510	39
Sourdough Breakfast Sandwich w/ bacon	1 item	470	24	11	NA	305	680	39
Sourdough Breakfast Sandwich w/ ham	1 item	450	20	9	NA	270	950	39
Sourdough Breakfast Sandwich w/ sausage	1 item	610	37	16	NA	290	1040	39
Croissant Sunrise item	1 item	360	21	8	NA	245	470	27
Croissant Sunrise item w/ bacon	1 item	410	25	9	NA	255	610	27
Croissant Sunrise item w/ sausage	1 item	550	40	14	NA	285	970	27
Breakfast Burrito	1 item	560	32	11	NA	495	980	52
Breakfast Burger	1 item	830	47	15	NA	275	1580	65
Breakfast Quesadilla	1 item	390	18	5	NA	285	920	NA
Scrambled Egg Breakfast w/ bacon	1 meal	760	42	11	NA	500	1140	NA
Scrambled Egg Breakfast w/ sausage	1 meal	900	56	15	NA	525	1480	NA
Low Carb Breakfast Bowl	11 oz.	900	73	33	NA	875	2050	NA
French Toast Dips w/o syrup	6 items	450	20	8	NA	5	570	58
Hash Brown Nuggets	4 oz.	330	21	5	NA	0	470	32

Carl's Jr.®
Continued

Burgers	Serving	Calories	Total fat (gm)	Saturated fat (gm)	Trans fats (gm)	Cholesterol (mg)	Sodium (mg)	Carbs (gm)
Hamburger	1 item	280	9	4	NA	35	480	NA
Big Hamburger	1 item	470	17	6	NA	60	1060	54
Famous Star Hamburger	1 item	590	32	9	NA	70	910	54
Famous Star w/ cheese	1 item	650	37	12	NA	85	1170	53
Six Dollar Burger	1 item	1000	62	25	NA	135	1690	60
Bacon Cheese Six Dollar Burger	1 item	1070	76	30	NA	170	1910	50
Guacamole Bacon Six Dollar Burger	1 item	1140	85	29	NA	160	2010	54
Low Carb Six Dollar Burger	1 item	490	37	16	NA	130	1270	6
Western Bacon Six Dollar Burger	1 item	1060	61	27	NA	135	2180	83
Chili Burger	1 item	690	35	15	NA	110	1400	NA
Jalapeno Burger	1 item	720	45	8	NA	90	1320	50
Kids Hamburger	1 item	460	17	6	NA	60	1060	53
Philly Cheesesteak Burger	1 item	830	55	17	NA	125	1510	52
Super Star Hamburger	1 item	790	47	14	NA	130	980	NA
Super Star w/ double cheese	1 item	920	57	21	NA	160	1490	54
Western Bacon Cheeseburger	1 item	660	30	12	NA	85	1410	70
Double Western Bacon Cheesburger	1 item	920	50	21	NA	155	1730	71
Sourdough Bacon Cheeseburger	1 item	550	29	14	NA	85	500	NA
Double Sourdough Bacon Cheeseburger	1 item	920	59	24	NA	170	1020	NA
Sandwich Items								
Charbroiled BBQ Chicken	1 item	370	4	1	NA	60	1070	48
Charbroiled Chicken Club	1 item	550	23	7	NA	95	1330	43
Charbroiled Santa Fe Chicken	1 item	610	32	8	NA	100	1440	43
Carl's Ranch Crispy Chicken	1 item	660	31	7	NA	70	1180	NA
Bacon Swiss Crispy Chicken	1 item	750	28	11	NA	80	1900	64
Western Bacon Crispy Chicken	1 item	760	38	11	NA	90	1550	NA
Spicy Chicken	1 item	460	26	5	NA	40	1220	59
Carl's Catch Fish item	1 item	560	27	7	NA	80	990	59
Fish n' Chips	1 item	630	28	5	NA	10	990	68
Baked Potatoes								
Potato w/o margarine	1 item	280	0	0	NA	0	30	NA
Potato w/ margarine	1 item	360	12	2	NA	0	140	NA
Broccoli & Cheese	1 item	510	21	5	NA	15	940	NA
Bacon & Cheese	1 item	620	29	8	NA	40	1160	NA
Sour Cream & Chive	1 item	410	14	4	NA	10	190	NA
Salads (w/o dressing)								
Charbroiled Chicken Salad-To-Go	1 salad	330	7	4	NA	75	680	16

Carl's Jr.®
Continued

Salads (w/o dressing) continued

	Serving	Calories	Total fat (gm)	Saturated fat (gm)	Trans fats (gm)	Cholesterol (mg)	Sodium (mg)	Carbs (gm)
Garden Salad-To-Go	1 salad	120	3	2	NA	5	230	5
Buffalo Ranch Chicken Salad	1 salad	380	16	3	NA	35	1180	NA
Sides								
French Fries (small)	3.5 oz.	290	14	3	NA	0	170	37
CrissCut Fries	5 oz.	410	24	5	NA	0	950	43
Chili Cheese Fries	12 oz.	920	51	16	NA	65	1030	NA
Onion Rings	4.5 oz.	440	22	5	NA	0	700	53
Zucchini	5 oz.	320	19	5	NA	0	680	31
Chicken Stars	6 pieces	270	17	5	NA	40	500	14
Chicken Breast Strip	3 pieces	360	21	4	NA	55	1360	NA
Shakes								
Chocolate Shake (small)	21 fl. oz.	540	11	7	NA	45	360	85
Strawberry Shake (small)	21 fl. oz.	520	11	7	NA	45	340	84
Vanilla Shake (small)	21 fl. oz.	470	11	7	NA	45	350	86

Carrabba's Italian Grills®
Does not provide nutrition information.

Cheesecake Factory®
Does not provide nutrition information.

NOTES:

_____

_____

_____

_____

_____

_____

_____

_____

_____

_____

Chick-fil-A®

	Serving	Calories	Total fat (gm)	Saturated fat (gm)	Trans fats (gm)	Cholesterol (mg)	Sodium (mg)	Carbs (gm)
Breakfast								
Chick-fil-A Chicken Biscuit	1 item	400	18	5	3	30	1200	44
Chick-fil-A Chicken Biscuit w/ cheese	1 item	450	23	7	3	45	1430	44
Chick-n-Minis	3 pieces	280	11	4	1	45	580	29
Chicken Biscuit	1 item	420	19	5	3	35	1270	44
Chicken, Egg, & Cheese on Sunflower Bagel	1 item	500	20	7	0	290	1260	49
Cinnamon Cluster	1 item	400	15	6	0	35	280	61
Biscuit w/ bacon	1 item	300	14	4	3	5	780	NA
Biscuit w/ bacon & egg	1 item	390	20	6	3	250	860	39
Biscuit w/ bacon, egg & cheese	1 item	430	24	9	3	265	1070	39
Biscuit w/ egg	1 item	340	16	5	3	245	740	NA
Biscuit w/ egg & cheese	1 item	390	21	7	3	260	960	NA
Biscuit w/ sausage	1 item	410	23	9	3	20	740	38
Biscuit w/ sausge & egg	1 item	500	29	11	3	265	810	NA
Biscuit w/ sausage, egg & cheese	1 item	540	33	13	3	280	1030	39
Biscuit w/ gravy	6.75 oz.	310	13	4	3	5	930	43
Breakfast Burritto Chicken	1 item	410	16	7	0	210	940	42
Breakfast Burritto Sausage	1 item	450	23	9	0	215	860	39
Hashbrowns	3 oz.	170	9	5	2	10	350	25
Sunflower Multigrain Bagel	1 item	220	3	0	0	0	350	NA
Sandwiches								
Chicken Sandwich	1 item	410	16	4	0	60	1300	38
Chicken Deluxe Sandwich	1 item	420	16	4	0	60	1300	NA
Chargrilled Chicken Sandwich	1 item	270	4	1	0	65	940	33
Chargrilled Chicken Club w/o sauce	1 item	380	11	0	0	90	1240	33
Cool Wraps								
Chargrilled Cool Wrap	1 wrap	390	7	3	0	65	1020	46
Caeser Cool Wrap	1 wrap	460	10	6	0	80	1350	44
Spicy Chicken Cool Wrap	1 wrap	380	6	3	0	60	1090	44
Specialties								
Chick Strips	4 items	290	13	3	0	65	730	15
Chicken Nuggets	8 items	260	12	3	0	70	1090	10
Chicken Salad on Whole Wheat	1 item	350	15	3	0	65	880	32
Breast of Chicken Soup	8.5 oz.	140	4	1	0	25	900	18
Side Items & Salads								
Waffle Potato Fries (small)	3 oz.	280	14	5	0	15	105	34
Southwest Chargrilled Salad w/o dressing	1 salad	240	8	4	0	60	770	17

Chick-fil-A®
Continued
Side Items & Salads continued

	Serving	Calories	Total fat (gm)	Saturated fat (gm)	Trans fats (gm)	Cholesterol (mg)	Sodium (mg)	Carbs (gm)
Chargrilled Chicken Salad w/o dressing	1 salad	180	6	3	0	65	620	9
Chick Strips Salad w/o dressing	1 salad	390	18	5	0	80	860	21
Chicken Salad Cup	1 item	270	18	3	0	85	790	8
Hearty Breast of Chicken Soup	1 item	140	4	1	0	25	900	18
Side Salad w/o dressing	1 salad	60	3	2	0	10	75	NA
Carrot & Raisin Salad (small)	4 oz.	170	6	1	0	10	110	28
Cole Slaw	4.5 oz.	260	21	4	0	25	220	17
Fresh Fruit Cup	4 oz.	60	0	0	0	0	0	13

Fast Food Factoid:

Way to go Chick-fil-A! Chick-fil-A does not use trans fats to fry any of its fried foods. This is one of two places where french fries are coded GREEN. Tell your friends. The other place is In-N-Out Burger, with locations in California, Nevada, and Arizona.

Chili's®
Starters

	Serving	Calories	Total fat (gm)	Saturated fat (gm)	Trans fats (gm)	Cholesterol (mg)	Sodium (mg)	Carbs (gm)
Awsome Blossom w/ dipping Sauce	1 order	2710	203	36	NA	NA	6360	194
Bottomless Tostada Chips	1 order	400	36	6	NA	NA	1540	18
Chicken Crispers	1 order	780	63	11	NA	NA	1390	21
Classic Nachos	1 order	1450	108	57	NA	NA	2730	53
Fried Cheese	1 order	1210	89	28	NA	NA	2470	82
Hot Spinach & Artichoke Dip W/ Tostada Chips	1 order	905	36	5	NA	NA	1560	74
Skillet Queso w/ Tostada Chips	1 order	1070	89	37	NA	NA	3920	30
Southwest Eggrolls w/ dipping sauce	1 order	810	51	10	NA	NA	1250	59
Texas Cheese Fries w/ Dressing	1 order	2070	160	73	NA	NA	3730	73
Wings Over Buffalo w/ dressing	1 order	1140	100	22	NA	NA	2540	4

Salads w/ dressing

	Serving	Calories	Total fat (gm)	Saturated fat (gm)	Trans fats (gm)	Cholesterol (mg)	Sodium (mg)	Carbs (gm)
Boneless Buffalo Chicken Salad	1 salad	910	58	13	NA	NA	620	51
Caesar Salad w/ Chicken & Dressing	1 salad	1010	76	13	NA	NA	1910	39
Caesar Salad w/ Shrimp & Dressing	1 salad	980	77	13	NA	NA	1900	39

Chili's®
Continued

Salads w/ dressing continued

	Serving	Calories	Total fat (gm)	Saturated fat (gm)	Trans fats (gm)	Cholesterol (mg)	Sodium (mg)	Carbs (gm)
Crispy Chicken Salad	1 salad	1250	87	13	NA	NA	2550	NA
Dinner Salad-House	1 salad	140	7	3	NA	NA	190	12
Lettuce Wraps w/ Dipping Sauce	1 salad	580	35	5	NA	NA	2330	55
Mesquite Chicken Salad	1 salad	800	43	16	NA	NA	2600	53
Southwest Cobb Salad	1 salad	1160	61	15	NA	NA	3830	56
Grilled Caribbean Salad	1 salad	710	32	5	NA	NA	1740	51
Quesadilla Explosion	1 item	1240	84	27	NA	NA	2660	81

Items

	Serving	Calories	Total fat (gm)	Saturated fat (gm)	Trans fats (gm)	Cholesterol (mg)	Sodium (mg)	Carbs (gm)
Cajun Chicken item	1 item	820	43	11	NA	NA	2220	66
Chicken Ranch Sandwich	1 item	1150	70	11	NA	NA	2830	82
Chili's Cheesesteak	1 item	1010	55	24	NA	NA	2510	77
Grilled Chicken	1 item	840	47	12	NA	NA	1950	57
Pita-Chicken Caesar	1 item	650	41	7	NA	NA	1540	31
Pita-Chicken Fajita	1 item	450	17	3	NA	NA	1750	35
Pita-Steak Fajita	1 item	580	33	10	NA	NA	1770	32
Smoked Turkey Sandwich	1 item	930	57	15	NA	NA	2920	65
Smoked Turkey Sandwich w/ Bacon	1 item	1030	64	18	NA	NA	3290	66

Big Mouth Burgers

	Serving	Calories	Total fat (gm)	Saturated fat (gm)	Trans fats (gm)	Cholesterol (mg)	Sodium (mg)	Carbs (gm)
Bacon Burger	1 item	1080	71	22	NA	NA	1660	54
BBQ Ranch Burger	1 item	1110	71	22	NA	NA	1920	60
Chipotle Bleu Cheese Bacon Burger	1 item	1090	71	21	NA	NA	2070	57
Ground Peppercorn Burger	1 item	1050	68	17	NA	NA	1410	61
Oldtimer	1 item	800	44	13	NA	NA	1190	54
Mushroom & Swiss	1 item	1100	71	21	NA	NA	1590	60

Chili's Grill

	Serving	Calories	Total fat (gm)	Saturated fat (gm)	Trans fats (gm)	Cholesterol (mg)	Sodium (mg)	Carbs (gm)
Margarita Grilled Chicken	1 order	690	14	3	NA	NA	2980	81
Cajun Ribeye Steak	1 order	870	76	28	NA	NA	730	3
Classic Sirloin Steak	1 order	540	42	14	NA	NA	820	1
Citrus Fire Chicken & Shrimp	1 order	760	27	5	NA	NA	2990	34
Grilled Baby Back Ribs	1 order	1370	82	24	NA	NA	4410	33
Monterey Chicken	1 order	1170	71	29	NA	NA	3530	67
Grilled Salmon w/ garlic & herbs	1 order	700	33	8	NA	NA	1420	53

Guiltless Grill

	Serving	Calories	Total fat (gm)	Saturated fat (gm)	Trans fats (gm)	Cholesterol (mg)	Sodium (mg)	Carbs (gm)
Chicken item	1 item	490	8	2	NA	NA	2720	63
Chicken Platter	1 order	580	9	3	NA	NA	2780	85
Pita	1 item	550	9	3	NA	NA	2110	NA
Tomato Basil Pasta	1 order	650	14	3	NA	NA	2560	NA

Chili's®
Continued

Guiltless Grill continued	Serving	Calories	Total fat (gm)	Saturated fat (gm)	Trans fats (gm)	Cholesterol (mg)	Sodium (mg)	Carbs (gm)
Salmon	1 order	480	14	3	NA	NA	1080	31
Black Bean Burger	1 item	650	12	2	NA	NA	1940	41
Fajitas								
Classic-Beef w/o toppings boat	3 items	1160	59	22	NA	NA	4210	20
Classic-Chicken w/o toppings boat	3 items	700	21	6	NA	NA	3050	23
Toppings Boat	1 order	240	19	10	NA	NA	310	8
Favorites								
Cajun Chicken Pasta	1 order	1460	75	38	NA	NA	5800	123
Chicken Tacos	1 order	1200	41	19	NA	NA	4620	126
Grilled Shrimp Alfredo	1 order	1340	72	37	NA	NA	5120	123
Chicken Crispers	1 order	1970	129	25	NA	NA	3020	133
Fajita Quesadillas–Beef w/o guacamole	1 order	1970	106	53	NA	NA	5580	151
Fajita Quesadillas–Chicken w/o guacamole	1 order	1720	82	44	NA	NA	5000	151
Guacamole	1 order	50	5	1	NA	NA	110	3
Tomato Basil Chicken Pasta	1 order	860	26	5	NA	NA	3980	NA
Country Fried Steak	1 order	1890	107	29	NA	NA	2750	148
Just For Kids								
Cheese Pizza	1 order	570	24	10	NA	NA	1130	67
Corn Dog	1 order	250	17	4	NA	NA	260	18
Grilled Cheese Sandwich	1 order	420	27	16	NA	NA	1200	26
Grilled Chicken Platter	1 order	140	3	1	NA	NA	790	3
Grilled Chicken Sandwich	1 order	170	3	1	NA	NA	670	16
Kraft Macaroni & Cheese	1 order	510	18	6	NA	NA	940	69
Little Chicken Crispers	1 order	590	42	8	NA	NA	1300	19
Little Mouth Burger	1 item	180	15	5	NA	NA	300	14
Little Mouth Cheeseburger	1 item	350	21	9	NA	NA	600	14
Pepper Pals Pasta w/ Alfredo Sauce	1 item	410	17	9	NA	NA	1680	47
Pepper Pals Pasta w/ Marinara Sauce	1 item	290	5	1	NA	NA	1510	52
Ribs Basket	1 item	370	24	9	NA	NA	1960	16
Side Items								
Mashed Potatoes w/ pepper gravy	1 order	450	28	7	NA	NA	1080	44
Homestyle Fries	1 order	430	26	5	NA	NA	250	53
Steamed Broccoli	1 order	80	6	1	NA	NA	280	6
Sautéed Mushrooms, Onions, Bell Peppers	1 order	120	10	2	NA	NA	360	6
Fresh Veggies	1 order	90	6	1	NA	NA	90	8

Chipotle Mexican Grill®

Items

Items	Serving	Calories	Total fat (gm)	Saturated fat (gm)	Trans fats (gm)	Cholesterol (mg)	Sodium (mg)	Carbs (gm)
13" Flour Tortillas	1 items	330	8	3	NA	0	710	NA
6" Flour Tortillas	3 items	300	8	3	NA	0	630	NA
Crispy Taco Shell	4 items	240	9	2	NA	0	40	NA
Rice	5 oz.	240	7	1	NA	0	610	NA
Black Beans	4 oz.	130	1	1	NA	0	318	NA
Pinto Beans	4 oz.	138	1	1	NA	0	374	NA
Fajita Vegetables	3 oz.	100	8	1	NA	0	640	NA
Barbacoa	5 oz.	285	16	4	NA	74	680	NA
Carnitas	4 oz.	227	12	3	NA	66	873	NA
Chicken	4 oz.	219	11	2	NA	96	431	NA
Steak	4 oz.	230	12	4	NA	51	306	NA
Tomato Salsa	4 oz.	25	0	0	NA	0	560	NA
Corn Salsa	4 oz.	100	1	0	NA	0	540	NA
Red Tomatillo	2 oz.	28	1	0	NA	0	493	NA
Green Tomatillo	2 oz.	15	1	0	NA	0	227	NA
Cheese	1 oz.	110	9	6	NA	30	180	NA
Sour Cream	2 oz.	120	10	7	NA	40	30	NA
Guacamole	4 oz.	170	15	3	NA	0	370	NA
Lettuce	1 oz.	5	0	0	NA	0	0	NA
Chips	4 oz.	490	19	4	NA	0	130	NA
Vinaigrette	2 oz.	282	26	3	NA	17	1525	NA

Fast Food Factoid:

Preventing common chronic diseases and premature death later in life requires that you take action now, even though you have no symptoms of chronic diseases. Look for the GREEN foods.

Chuck E. Cheese®

	Serving	Calories	Total fat (gm)	Saturated fat (gm)	Trans fats (gm)	Cholesterol (mg)	Sodium (mg)	Carbs (gm)
Appetizers								
Italian Bread Sticks	1 item	193	8	1	NA	2	370	27
Buffalo Wings	12 items	660	45	10	NA	330	1680	3
Mozzarella Sticks	1 item	105	6	2	NA	10	256	7
Pizza (medium)								
All Meat Combo	1 slice	292	12	4	NA	26	738	33
BBQ Chicken	1 slice	269	8	3	NA	21	651	43
Cheese	1 slice	237	7	3	NA	14	542	33
Pepperoni	1 slice	263	10	4	NA	19	632	33
Pepperoni & Sausage	1 slice	281	11	4	NA	23	686	33
Canadian Bacon & Pineapple	1 slice	245	7	3	NA	15	608	34
Vegetarian	1 slice	237	7	3	NA	13	543	36
Items & Side Items								
Hot Dog	1 item	170	17	6	NA	40	830	27
Ham & Cheese	1 item	672	28	7	NA	68	2296	70
Italian Sub	1 item	792	40	12	NA	83	2503	69
Grilled Chicken Club	1 item	652	31	9	NA	98	1936	70
French Fries	5 oz.	241	9	0	NA	0	411	37
Birthday Cake White or Chocolate								
1 of 10 Slices	1 slice	310	13	4	NA	30	490	45

Fast Food Factoid:

Rome wasn't built in a single day and a lifetime of eating habits can't be altered overnight. Choose just one GREEN food...you have to start sometime.

NOTES:

_____

_____

_____

_____

Church's®

Main Course	Serving	Calories	Total fat (gm)	Saturated fat (gm)	Trans fats (gm)	Cholesterol (mg)	Sodium (mg)	Carbs (gm)
Original Wing	1 item	300	19	5	3	120	540	7
Original Leg	1 item	110	6	2	1	55	280	3
Original Thigh	1 item	330	23	6	3	110	680	8
Original Breast	1 item	200	11	3	2	80	450	3
Spicy Wing	1 item	430	27	7	4	125	1020	17
Spicy Leg	1 item	180	11	3	2	65	470	8
Spicy Thigh	1 item	480	35	9	5	135	1035	20
Spicy Breast	1 item	320	20	5	4	75	760	12
Bigger Better Chicken Sandwich w/ Cheese	1 item	510	27	7	2	50	1070	46
Spicy Chicken Sandwich	1 item	360	18	4	1.5	30	660	NA
Original Tender Strips	1 piece	120	6	2	1	35	440	6
Spicy Tender Strips	1 piece	135	7	2	2	25	480	7
Country Fried Steak w/ gravy	1 piece	470	28	7	NA	65	1620	36
Sides								
Honey Butter Biscuits	1 item	250	16	4	NA	5	640	28
Mashed Potatoes & Gravy	Regular	70	2	0	0	1	480	12
Okra	Regular	300	23	4	NA	0	740	36
Corn on the Cob	1 ear	140	3	0	NA	0	15	24
Country Fried Steak Sandwich	1 item	490	32	8	2	30	880	36
Whole Jalapeño Peppers	2 items	10	0	0	0	0	390	NA
Cole Slaw	Regular	150	10	2	0	5	170	15
French Fries	Regular	420	20	6	6	5	450	38
Cajun Rice	Regular	130	7	3	0	5	260	16
Jalapeño Bombers	4 items	240	10	6	NA	30	970	29
Sweet Corn Nuggets	Regular	600	29	2	NA	0	1260	72
Collard Greens	Regular	25	0	0	0	0	170	5
Macaroni & Cheese	Regular	210	11	4	NA	15	690	23
Spicy Fish Sandwich	1 item	320	20	4	3	25	560	25
Spicy Fish Fillet	1 item	160	9	2	3	25	350	13
Desserts								
Edward's Double Lemon Pie	1 pie	300	14	6	NA	25	160	39
Edward's Strawberry Cream Cheese Pie	1 pie	280	15	8	NA	15	130	32
Apple Pie	1 pie	260	11	4	2	5	250	39

Cici's Pizza®
Pizza (buffet)

	Serving	Calories	Total fat (gm)	Saturated fat (gm)	Trans fats (gm)	Cholesterol (mg)	Sodium (mg)	Carbs (gm)
Alfredo Pizza	1 slice	139	5	3	1	10	199	18
Bar-B-Que Pizza	1 slice	172	6	4	1	12	311	18
Bacon Cheddar	1 slice	145	5	2	0	13	312	21
Beef Pizza	1 slice	169	7	4	1	20	281	18
Cheese Pizza	1 slice	152	5	3	1	9	305	20
Ham & Pineapple	1 slice	141	4	3	1	10	319	19
Olé Pizza	1 slice	107	4	2	1	1	261	13
Pepperoni & Jalapeño Pizza	1 slice	163	6	4	1	11	394	20
Pepperoni Pizza	1 slice	175	7	4	1	13	384	20
Sausage Pizza	1 slice	197	7	4	1	11	358	19
Spinach Alfredo Pizza	1 slice	150	5	3	1	11	215	20
Zesty Ham & Cheddar Pizza	1 slice	152	6	3	1	9	271	18
Zesty Pepperoni Pizza	1 slice	156	7	3	1	7	302	18
Zesty Tomato Alfredo Pizza	1 slice	136	5	3	1	10	202	18
Zesty Veggie Pizza	1 slice	124	4	2	1	3	224	17

Cracker Barrel Old Country Store®

Does not provide nutrition information, but here is a list of some of their healthier options.

Turkey sausage is offered as an alternative to regular sausage.

Entrée salads are available on the menu.

Promise spread is available as an alternative to butter.

Eggstrod'naire is available on the breakfast menu.

Oatmeal is available on the menu.

Apple Bran Muffins are available as a bread choice.

Decaffeinated Hot Tea & Coffee are available as additional beverages.

Fresh Bananas & Raisins are available.

Special K, Wheaties, and Cheerios are included in the dry cereal offering.

Sweet & Low, Splenda, and Equal are available on each table.

Low Calorie Fruit Spread is available.

Sugar Free Maple Syrup is available.

Boiled Chicken Tenders are not printed on the menu, but are available upon request.

No Sugar Added Apple Pie & No Sugar Added Vanilla Ice Cream are available.

Culver's®

	Serving	Calories	Total fat (gm)	Saturated fat (gm)	Trans fats (gm)	Cholesterol (mg)	Sodium (mg)	Carbs (gm)
Burgers								
Cheddar Burger	1 item	641	37	18	1	160	750	31
Chicken Salad Wrap	1 item	518	26	7	0	83	1133	39
Butterburger, Single	1 item	346	15	6	1	65	690	35
Butterburger, Double	1 item	480	23	9	1	120	720	36
Butterburger, Single w/ cheese	1 item	398	20	8	1	78	945	36
Butterburger, Double w/ cheese	1 item	580	32	14	1	145	1230	37
Butterburger, Single w/ bacon	1 item	586	39	12	1	103	1048	34
Butterburger, Double w/ bacon	1 item	764	51	18	1	170	1332	34
Butterburger, Single Deluxe	1 item	507	32	10	1	88	838	34
Butterburger, Double Deluxe	1 item	684	44	15	1	155	1042	34
Butterburger, Low Carb	1 item	443	32	14	1	150	862	1
Grilled Reuben Melt	1 item	608	31	13	1	112	1930	43
Mushroom & Swiss Burger	1 item	680	31	14	1	146	1143	60
Sourdough Melt	1 item	586	31	13	1	145	1040	37
Tuna Salad on Grilled Sourdough	1 item	484	25	7	0	56	1008	34
Wisconsin Swiss Melt	1 item	575	30	13	1	146	980	36
Other Items								
Beef Frank on a Bun	1 item	412	25	10	1	40	1471	38
Cheese Dog	1 item	481	34	15	NA	70	1270	NA
Chili Dog	1 item	399	27	11	1	48	1250	28
Chili Cheese Dog	1 item	509	36	16	NA	78	1430	NA
Beef Pot Roast item	1 item	307	10	3	1	32	820	33
Crispy Chicken Filet item	1 item	614	27	6	0	60	1593	68
Homestyle Crispy Chicken Fillet item	1 item	620	28	6	NA	65	1763	68
Hot 'n Spicy Chicken item	1 item	452	17	3	NA	80	1193	NA
Grilled Chicken Breast item	1 item	370	8	3	0	70	1457	47
Roasted Grilled Chicken Breast Fillet item	1 item	375	8	3	NA	85	1407	47
Grilled Ham 'n Swiss on Rye	1 item	457	22	10	0	112	2212	35
North Atlantic Cod Fillet item	1 item	740	42	11	1	74	1239	58
Philly Ribeye Steak item	1 item	486	19	10	NA	78	1125	NA
Pork Tenderloin item	1 item	703	29	11	3	65	1641	87
Turkey Sourdough BLT	1 item	595	34	11	0	104	2089	39
Stacked Turkey item	1 item	463	20	4	0	66	1623	47
Daily Features								
Bacon, Lettuce & Tomato	1 item	507	32	9	NA	50	1038	NA
BBQ Chicken	1 item	337	11	3	NA	63	1186	NA
BBQ Pork	1 item	392	14	4	NA	51	1099	NA
Beef Franks Sauerkraut	1 item	357	22	8	1	50	1440	NA

Culver's® Continued

Daily Features continued

	Serving	Calories	Total fat (gm)	Saturated fat (gm)	Trans fats (gm)	Cholesterol (mg)	Sodium (mg)	Carbs (gm)
Beef Pot Roast Platter	1 item	928	40	13	1	99	2382	NA
Chicken Salad on Grilled Sourdough	1 item	555	29	8	0	101	1127	NA
Deli Dog	1 item	441	29	12	NA	51	1326	NA
Ham Reuben	1 item	501	24	10	NA	117	2532	NA
Grilled Pork Tenderloin	1 item	581	22	5	NA	95	1173	NA
Pork Tenderloin	1 item	568	21	9	0	100	1192	NA
Stuffed Taco	1 taco	417	22	9	NA	39	667	NA
Turkey Reuben	1 item	396	14	5	NA	74	1995	NA
Western Barbeque Beef	1 item	370	13	4	NA	48	820	NA

Dinners (includes fries, coleslaw & dinner roll)

	Serving	Calories	Total fat (gm)	Saturated fat (gm)	Trans fats (gm)	Cholesterol (mg)	Sodium (mg)	Carbs (gm)
Breaded Shrimp	1 meal	1264	55	17	0	215	3387	148
Chicken	1 meal	1684	90	25	1	325	3287	140
Fish 'n Chips	6 item	1152	64	20	3	64	1025	104
North Atlantic Cod Fillet	2 item	1461	84	23	1	118	1976	135

Kid's Meal (entrée only)

	Serving	Calories	Total fat (gm)	Saturated fat (gm)	Trans fats (gm)	Cholesterol (mg)	Sodium (mg)	Carbs (gm)
Butterburger	1 item	346	15	6	NA	65	690	35
Cheeseburger	1 item	396	20	8	NA	78	945	36
Corn Dog	1 item	260	14	4	NA	35	540	26
Hot Dog w/ bun	1 item	386	25	10	NA	40	1340	30
Grill Cheese on Sourdough	1 item	320	15	7	NA	35	900	36
French Fries (Jr.)	3.5 oz.	260	13	6	NA	0	105	38

Garden Fresh Salads (w/o dressing)

	Serving	Calories	Total fat (gm)	Saturated fat (gm)	Trans fats (gm)	Cholesterol (mg)	Sodium (mg)	Carbs (gm)
Avocado Pecan Bleu w/ Chicken	1 salad	557	41	11	0	78	1339	16
Chicken Cashew w/ Grilled Chicken	1 salad	441	25	8	0	105	1135	17
Cobb Salad	1 salad	531	31	11	0	135	2026	NA
Side	1 salad	100	6	3	0	15	163	6
Club	1 salad	455	24	10	0	112	2291	NA
Crispy Chicken Parmesan	1 salad	336	13	4	1	51	1096	34
Garden Salad	1 salad	163	9	5	NA	30	201	25
Hot 'n Spicy Chicken	1 salad	359	17	9	NA	100	1139	NA
Grilled Chicken Caesar	1 salad	308	12	4	NA	82	1298	15
Tossed Chicken	1 salad	515	34	11	0	116	1196	NA
Tossed Tuna	1 salad	399	25	6	0	42	770	NA

Soups

	Serving	Calories	Total fat (gm)	Saturated fat (gm)	Trans fats (gm)	Cholesterol (mg)	Sodium (mg)	Carbs (gm)
Bean w/ ham	10.5 oz.	205	3	1	0	7	1343	33
Chicken & Dumpling	10.5 oz.	306	22	9	3	60	1343	19
Chicken Gumbo	10.5 oz.	141	6	2	0	26	1420	13
Cream of Broccoli	10.5 oz.	185	10	5	0	33	1573	16

Culver's® Continued

Soups continued

	Serving	Calories	Total fat (gm)	Saturated fat (gm)	Trans fats (gm)	Cholesterol (mg)	Sodium (mg)	Carbs (gm)
Creamy Garden Vegetable	10 oz.	188	11	4	1	33	1693	19
George's Chili	10.5 oz.	336	18	6	0	66	1494	27
Tomato Florentine	10.5 oz.	120	1	0	0	0	1410	21
Vegetable Beef & Barley	10.5 oz.	120	4	1	0	13	1383	14
Side Items								
French Fries (regular)	5 oz.	364	18	9	0	0	147	53
Chili Cheddar Fries	9.5 oz.	634	35	18	0	46	689	73
Onion Rings	1 order	580	29	9	0	0	1070	70
Cole Slaw	5.5 oz.	350	21	4	0	25	690	37
Dinner Roll	1 roll	120	5	2	0	10	200	19
Mashed Potatoes & Gravy	7 oz.	152	3	0	0	2	394	26
Buffalo Chicken Tenders	4 items	392	19	4	NA	60	2200	NA
Breaded Chicken Tenders	4 items	420	18	6	NA	80	1152	32
Wisconsin Dairyland Cheese Curds	1 item	670	38	15	2	75	1740	54

Fast Food Factoid:

Taste, cost, and convenience are the main reasons many people struggle to eat good fast foods. Try a GREEN food—you might be surprised.

NOTES:

_____

_____

_____

_____

Dairy Queen®

	Serving	Calories	Total fat (gm)	Saturated fat (gm)	Trans fats (gm)	Cholesterol (mg)	Sodium (mg)	Carbs (gm)
Hamburgers								
DQ Homestyle Burger	1 item	290	12	5	0	45	630	33
DQ Homestyle Cheeseburger	1 item	340	17	8	0	55	850	34
DQ Homestyle Dbl Cheeseburger	1 item	540	31	16	0	115	1130	34
DQ Homestyle Bacon Double Cheeseburger	1 item	610	36	18	0	130	1380	35
DQ Ultimate Burger	1 item	670	43	19	0	135	1210	33
Flame Thrower Burger	1 item	810	60	22	0	160	1390	41
Classic Grillburger	1 item	540	30	11	3	65	990	42
Classic Grillburger w/ cheese	1 item	610	36	15	4	85	1110	42
½ lb. Grillburger	1 item	800	50	21	5	130	1230	42
½ lb. Grillburger w/ cheese	1 item	930	60	27	5	160	1380	47
Bacon Cheese Grillburger	1 item	710	45	19	4	105	1430	41
Mushroom Swiss Grillburger	1 item	700	47	16	4	90	890	39
California Grillburger	1 item	630	42	13	3	75	820	NA
Side & Other Items								
Hot Dog	1 item	240	14	5	0	25	730	30
Chili 'n Cheese Dog	1 item	330	21	9	0	45	1090	24
Crispy Chicken item	1 item	590	34	6	2	40	1100	47
Grilled Chicken item	1 item	340	16	3	0	55	1000	49
Chicken Strip Basket	4 item	920	49	9	12	40	2090	105
French Fries	4 oz.	300	12	3	4	0	700	50
Onion Rings	4 oz.	470	30	6	7	0	740	45
Salads								
Crispy Chicken Salad (no dressing)	1 salad	420	22	7	2	70	960	90
Grilled Chicken Salad (no dressing)	1 salad	270	11	5	0	80	1160	92
Side Salad (no dressing)	1 salad	45	0	0	0	0	50	27
Cones & Sundaes								
Chocolate Cone (small)	5 fl. oz.	240	8	5	0	20	115	22
Vanilla Cone (small)	5 fl. oz.	230	7	5	0	20	115	22
Dipped Cone (small)	5.5 fl. oz.	340	17	9	1	20	130	36
Chocolate Sundae (small)	6 fl. oz.	280	7	5	0	20	140	49
Strawberry Sundae (small)	6 fl. oz.	240	7	5	0	20	110	50
Royal Treats								
Banana Split	1 item	510	12	8	0	30	180	98
Brownie Earthquake	1 item	740	27	16	3	50	350	149
Peanut Buster Parfait	1 item	730	31	17	0	35	400	96
Triple Chocolate Utopia	1 item	770	39	17	2	55	390	NA
Strawberry Shortcake	1 item	430	14	9	1	60	360	NA

Dairy Queen®
Continued

Novelties & Blizzards

	Serving	Calories	Total fat (gm)	Saturated fat (gm)	Trans fats (gm)	Cholesterol (mg)	Sodium (mg)	Carbs (gm)
DQ item	1 item	200	6	3	1	10	140	32
Chocolate Dilly Bar	1 item	220	13	10	1	15	85	24
Buster Bar	1 item	500	28	15	1	15	230	45
Starkiss	1 item	80	0	0	0	0	10	21
DQ Fudge Bar	1 item	50	0	0	0	0	70	13
DQ Vanilla Orange Bar	1 item	60	0	0	0	0	40	17
Lemon DQ Freez'r	½ cup	80	0	0	0	0	10	NA
Oreo Cookies Blizzard (small)	10 fl. oz.	570	21	10	3	40	430	83
Arctic Rush Slush	small	240	0	0	0	0	0	48
Banana Split Blizzard (small)	10.5 fl. oz.	460	14	9	0	40	210	73
Reese's Peanut Butter Cup Blizzard (small)	11 fl. oz.	600	21	16	0	40	220	87
Caramel MooLatte	16 fl. oz.	630	19	16	0	35	260	103
Cappuccino MooLatte	16 fl. oz.	500	18	15	0	30	170	73
Chocolate Malt	small	650	15	10	0	50	310	112
Chocolate Shake	small	560	14	9	0	45	280	95
French Vanilla MooLatte	16 fl. oz.	570	18	14	0	30	170	90
Mocha MooLatte	16 fl. oz.	590	23	15	0	30	200	84
Strawberry-CheeseQuake Blizzard (small)	10 fl. oz.	530	21	13	1	85	320	76

Del Taco®

Breakfast

	Serving	Calories	Total fat (gm)	Saturated fat (gm)	Trans fats (gm)	Cholesterol (mg)	Sodium (mg)	Carbs (gm)
Breakfast Burrito	1 item	250	11	6	NA	160	529	24
Egg & Cheese Burrito	1 item	450	24	13	NA	530	40	39
Macho Bacon & Egg Burrito	1 item	1030	60	20	NA	790	1760	NA
Maple Sausage Rollup	1 item	270	16	5	NA	50	420	NA
Steak & Egg Burrito	1 item	580	34	16	NA	560	1270	41
Bacon & Egg Quesadilla	1 item	450	23	12	NA	260	920	40
Hash Brown Sticks	2 items	250	19	1	NA	0	200	20
Shredded Beef Breakfast Burrito	1 item	785	33	11	NA	382	1340	41

Tacos

	Serving	Calories	Total fat (gm)	Saturated fat (gm)	Trans fats (gm)	Cholesterol (mg)	Sodium (mg)	Carbs (gm)
Taco	1 taco	160	10	4	NA	20	150	11
Soft Taco	1 taco	160	8	4	NA	20	330	16
Chicken Soft Taco	1 taco	210	12	4	NA	30	520	18
Crispy Shrimp Taco	1 taco	342	21	5	NA	60	961	NA
Big Fat Taco	1 taco	320	11	5	NA	35	680	39
Big Fat Steak Taco	1 taco	390	19	6	NA	45	960	38
Big Fat Chicken Taco	1 taco	340	13	4	NA	45	840	38

Del Taco®
Continued

Tacos continued

	Serving	Calories	Total fat (gm)	Saturated fat (gm)	Trans fats (gm)	Cholesterol (mg)	Sodium (mg)	Carbs (gm)
Ultimate Taco	1 taco	260	17	8	NA	50	470	NA
Steak Taco Del Carbon	1 taco	220	11	4	NA	30	680	19
Chicken Taco Del Carbon	1 taco	170	5	1	NA	30	530	19
Carnitas Taco	1 taco	170	6	2	NA	25	370	NA
Crispy Fish Taco	1 taco	290	16	3	NA	20	460	30
Shredded Beef Taco Del Carbon	1 taco	199	11	2	NA	28	277	17

Burritos

	Serving	Calories	Total fat (gm)	Saturated fat (gm)	Trans fats (gm)	Cholesterol (mg)	Sodium (mg)	Carbs (gm)
Half-Pound Green Burrito	1 item	430	12	9	NA	20	1690	59
Half-Pound Red Burrito	1 item	430	12	9	NA	20	1670	65
Bean & Cheese Green Burrito	1 item	280	8	5	NA	15	1030	38
Bean & Cheese Red Burrito	1 item	270	8	5	NA	15	1020	38
Del Beef Burrito	1 item	550	30	17	NA	90	1090	42
Deluxe Del Beef Burrito	1 item	590	33	19	NA	95	1110	45
Del Combo Burrito	1 item	530	22	13	NA	55	1680	61
Deluxe Combo Burrito	1 item	570	25	15	NA	60	1700	64
Del Classic Chicken Burrito	1 item	560	36	13	NA	70	1100	41
Macho Beef Burrito	1 item	1170	62	29	NA	190	2190	89
Macho Chicken Buritto	1 item	930	33	15	NA	100	2990	111
Macho Combo Burrito	1 item	1050	44	21	NA	115	2760	113
Spicy Chicken Burrito	1 item	480	16	10	NA	40	1850	66
Chicken Works Burrito	1 item	520	23	12	NA	65	1620	57
Shredded Beef Combo Burrito	1 item	815	30	8	NA	70	1653	61
Steak Works Burrito	1 item	590	31	16	NA	70	1820	58
Veggie Works Burrito	1 item	490	18	11	NA	25	1660	69
Carnitas Burrito	1 item	440	21	12	NA	70	1050	NA

Quesadillas

	Serving	Calories	Total fat (gm)	Saturated fat (gm)	Trans fats (gm)	Cholesterol (mg)	Sodium (mg)	Carbs (gm)
Cheddar Quesadilla	1 item	500	27	20	NA	75	860	39
Spicy Jack Quesadilla	1 item	490	26	17	NA	75	920	38
Chicken Cheddar Quesadilla	1 item	580	31	21	NA	104	1240	41
Jalapeno Bacon & Chicken Quesadilla	1 item	612	34	18	NA	126	1093	NA
Spicy Jack Chicken Quesadilla	1 item	570	30	16	NA	105	1300	40

Salads

	Serving	Calories	Total fat (gm)	Saturated fat (gm)	Trans fats (gm)	Cholesterol (mg)	Sodium (mg)	Carbs (gm)
Deluxe Chicken Salad w/ dressing	1 salad	740	34	15	NA	70	2610	77
Mexican Caesar Salad	1 salad	557	47	9	NA	14	444	16
Taco Salad w/ salsa & sour cream	1 salad	350	30	10	NA	45	390	10
Deluxe Taco Salad w/ salsa & sour cream	1 salad	780	40	18	NA	80	2250	76

Del Taco®
Continued

Burgers	Serving	Calories	Total fat (gm)	Saturated fat (gm)	Trans fats (gm)	Cholesterol (mg)	Sodium (mg)	Carbs (gm)
Hamburger	1 item	280	9	3	NA	25	640	37
Cheeseburger	1 item	330	13	6	NA	35	870	37
Del Cheeseburger	1 item	430	25	7	NA	45	710	35
Double Del Cheeseburger	1 item	560	35	12	NA	85	960	35
Bacon Double Del Cheeseburger	1 item	610	39	14		95	1130	35
Bun Taco	1 item	440	21	12	NA	65	830	37
Side Items								
Nachos	4 oz	380	24	8	NA	5	630	40
Macho Nachos	1 item	1100	63	24	NA	55	2640	113
Chips and Salsa	1 item	155	7	3	NA	0	290	22
French Fries (regular)	5 oz	350	23	4	NA	0	270	34
Chili Cheese Fries	10.5 oz	670	46	15	NA	45	880	51
Rice Cup	4 oz.	140	2	1	NA	2	910	27
Beans 'n Cheese Cup	8 oz.	260	3	2	NA	5	1810	47

Fast Food Factoid:

Despite the scientific evidence that supports the need to consume whole grains and cereals, food makers claim that Chocolate Frosted Sugar Bombs breakfast cereal is part of a healthy breakfast.

NOTES:

_____

_____

_____

_____

_____

_____

Denny's®

Breakfast Menu

	Serving	Calories	Total fat (gm)	Saturated fat (gm)	Trans fats (gm)	Cholesterol (mg)	Sodium (mg)	Carbs (gm)
Meat Lover's Breakfast	21 oz.	1027	60	18	0	497	3462	109
Original Grand Slam	11 oz.	665	49	15	0	515	1106	56
All American Slam w/ hash browns	14 oz.	990	78	27	1	830	2310	21
French Slam	2 slice	1196	83	29	0	789	2302	74
Grand Slam Slugger w/ hash brown	27 oz.	1190	57	16	0	480	3250	97
Meat Lover's Scramble	21 oz.	1241	72	21	0	557	5575	103
Heartland Scramble	22 oz.	1111	66	20	0	550	3197	118
Denver Scramble w/ hash browns	22 oz.	1090	50	15	0	551	3680	NA
Meat Lover's Bowl	25 oz.	1414	99	30	NA	547	2984	NA
Country Sausage Bowl	28 oz.	1427	99	29	NA	537	3543	NA
Ham & Mushroom Bowl	24 oz.	1304	90	26	NA	540	2632	NA
Lumberjack Slam w/ hash browns	22 oz.	1170	57	16	0	590	4200	108
Ultimate Omelette	12 oz.	619	50	16	1	770	1214	26
Veggie-Cheese Omelette	12 oz.	494	39	12	NA	747	719	28
Veggie-Cheese Omelette w/ EggBeaters	12 oz.	346	22	7	NA	23	849	11
Ham & Cheddar Omelette	10 oz.	595	47	16	1	783	1200	5
Ham & Cheddar Omelette w/ EggBeaters	10 oz.	468	32	11	NA	58	1351	5
Country Fried Steak & Eggs	8 oz.	464	34	9	0	527	828	49
T-Bone Steak & Eggs	14 oz.	991	77	31	0	657	1003	1
Steakhouse Strip & Eggs	11 oz.	662	48	24	0	624	895	3
Moons Over My Hammy	13 oz.	841	51	22	0.5	580	2699	52
Belgian Waffle Platter	8 oz.	619	45	22	0	274	1683	28
Fabulous French Toast Platter	3 slices	1261	79	30	0	422	2495	110
Fruit Filled Cherry Pancakes	18 oz.	909	55	15	NA	530	2432	NA
Fruit Filled Blueberry Pancakes	18 oz.	921	55	15	NA	530	2430	NA
Fruit Filled Apple Cinnamon Pancakes	19 oz.	924	56	15	NA	530	2498	NA
Buttermilk Pancake Platter	3 items	660	25	8	0	50	2530	83
Buttermilk Pancake	9 oz.	420	5	1	0	0	1350	82
Country Fried Potatoes	3 items	394	20	6	3	9	938	23
Hash Browns	4 oz.	197	12	2	0	0	446	20
Hash Browns w/ cheddar cheese	6 oz.	280	19	6	0	23	583	21
Hash Browns w/ onions, cheese, gravy	8 oz.	493	25	9	0	29	3534	54
Grits	4 oz.	80	0	0	0	0	520	18
Breakfast a la Carte								
One Egg	2 oz.	120	10	3	0	210	120	1
Two Eggs & More Breakfast	11 oz.	678	55	17	0	506	898	21

Denny's® Continued

Breakfast a la Carte continued

	Serving	Calories	Total fat (gm)	Saturated fat (gm)	Trans fats (gm)	Cholesterol (mg)	Sodium (mg)	Carbs (gm)
EggBeaters Egg Substitute	4 oz.	56	0	0	0	0	186	2
Ham, grilled slice, Honey smoked	3 oz.	85	3	2	0	49	1700	6
Bacon, 4 strips	4 strips	162	18	5	0	36	640	1
Sausage, 4 links	4 links	354	32	12	0	64	944	0
Sausage Patties	2 items	295	28	10	0	57	450	1
Toast, dry	1 slice	90	1	0	0	0	166	17
English Muffin, dry	1 item	125	1	0	0	0	198	27
Bagel, dry	1 item	310	1	0	0	0	640	65
Biscuit	2 oz.	192	10	2	4	1	519	22
Quaker Oatmeal	4 oz.	100	2	0	0	0	175	18
Kellogg's Dry Cereal	1 oz.	100	0	0	0	0	276	23
Musselman's Applesauce	3 oz.	60	0	0	0	0	13	15
Banana, whole	4 oz.	110	0	0	0	0	0	29
Grapefruit	½	60	0	0	0	0	0	16
Grapes	3 oz.	55	1	0	0	0	0	15

Fit Fare (contains less than 15 gm fat)

	Serving	Calories	Total fat (gm)	Saturated fat (gm)	Trans fats (gm)	Cholesterol (mg)	Sodium (mg)	Carbs (gm)
Slim Slam (w/o topping)	13 oz.	490	11	3	0	45	2160	76
Skinny Moons	15 oz.	650	14	3	0	45	1950	73
Veggie Egg Beaters Omelette w/ English muffin	14 oz.	330	8	3	0	0	850	37
Toast, dry	1 oz.	92	1	0	0	0	166	17
English Muffin, dry	2 oz.	150	2	0	0	0	230	27
Bagel, dry	4 oz.	310	1	0	0	0	640	65
Oatmeal	4 oz.	100	2	0	0	0	175	18
Grits	4 oz.	80	0	0	0	0	520	18
Cereal (average)	1 oz.	100	0	0	0	0	276	23
Grapes	3 oz.	55	1	0	0	0	0	15
Banana (1)	4 oz.	110	0	0	0	0	0	29
Apple Juice	10 oz.	126	0	0	0	0	24	33
Ruby Red Grapefruit Juice	10 oz.	162	0	0	0	0	43	41
Orange Juice	10 oz.	126	0	0	0	0	31	31
Tomato Juice	10 oz.	56	0	0	0	0	921	11
Boca Burger w/ small fruit bowl	15 oz.	508	11	3	0	15	1308	83
Turkey Breast Salad w/o dressing	13 oz.	230	10	5	0	45	1310	NA
Grilled Chicken Breast Salad	15 oz.	310	13	6	0	90	800	15
Side Garden Salad w/o dressing	7 oz.	113	7	5	0	0	144	6
Vegetable Beef Soup	8 oz.	79	1	1	0	5	820	18
Chicken Noodle	8 oz.	110	6	1	0	25	1130	15
Grilled Chicken Breast Dinner	11 oz.	190	3	1	0	70	650	12

Denny's® Continued

Fit Fare continued

	Serving	Calories	Total fat (gm)	Saturated fat (gm)	Trans fats (gm)	Cholesterol (mg)	Sodium (mg)	Carbs (gm)
Tilapia w/ rice, green beans & tomato slice	18 oz.	410	11	3	0	85	1270	40
Baked Potato, plain w/ skin	7 oz.	220	0	0	0	0	16	51
Mashed Potatoes	5 oz.	168	7	3	0	8	498	23
Corn	4 oz.	110	2	0	0	0	180	23
Green Beans	4 oz.	40	1	0	0	2	47	5
Musselman's Applesauce	3 oz.	60	0	0	0	0	13	15
Sliced Tomatoes	2 oz.	13	0	0	0	0	6	3

Promotional Items

	Serving	Calories	Total fat (gm)	Saturated fat (gm)	Trans fats (gm)	Cholesterol (mg)	Sodium (mg)	Carbs (gm)
Peach French Toast	16 oz.	1370	85	34	0	863	2385	NA
Zesty Creole Scrambles	24 oz.	1310	74	22	0	505	3810	NA
Ham & Jalapeño Scramble	25 oz.	1110	55	19	0	570	3930	NA
Pepper Jack & Small Sausage	27 oz.	1430	92	33	1	605	4270	NA
Pot Roast Dinner	7 oz.	266	16	6	0	94	873	NA
Chicken Fried Chicken Dinner	11 oz.	550	29	6	1	102	2621	NA
Tilapia w/ Creole sauce	14 oz.	490	23	5	0	90	1710	NA
Chicken Tangy Lemon Mushroom	14 oz.	660	43	15	1	185	1780	NA
Texas Style Steak Tips	15 oz.	700	40	10	0	90	2290	NA
Mushroom Swiss Chopped Steak	14 oz.	800	73	29	0	173	1140	NA
Hershey's Chocolate Cake	5 oz.	631	33	13	2	40	420	NA

Items, Salads & Soups

	Serving	Calories	Total fat (gm)	Saturated fat (gm)	Trans fats (gm)	Cholesterol (mg)	Sodium (mg)	Carbs (gm)
Club item	12 oz.	602	38	6	0	41	2450	39
The Super Bird item	10 oz.	479	29	11	0	47	1764	40
Grilled Chicken item w/o dressing	10 oz.	476	14	3	0	77	1494	57
Bacon, Lettuce & Tomato	7 oz.	610	38	9	0	35	862	50
Bacon Cheddar Burger	1 item	860	61	27	3	195	2070	33
BBQ Chicken item	17 oz.	1089	62	14	NA	103	1872	NA
Classic Burger	11 oz.	694	35	12	2.5	100	785	56
Classic Burger w/ cheese	13 oz.	852	48	20	2.5	140	1385	57
Chicken Ranch Melt	13 oz.	838	47	15	2.5	109	2481	84
Crispy Onion Burger w/ Fries	1 item	1640	105	29	3	170	1830	128
Jalapeno Burger w/ Fries	1 item	1480	93	28	3	170	1870	109
Philly Melt	18 oz.	874	50	16	2.5	114	2444	68
Italian Chicken Melt	21 oz.	1134	62	20	NA	115	3735	NA
Boca Burger	11 oz.	452	11	3	0	14	1290	64
Mushroom Swiss Burger	16 oz.	880	49	19	3.5	137	1619	63
Mini Burgers w/ Onion Rings	1 item	2220	136	31	0	179	3860	179
Western Burger w/ Fries	1 item	1500	84	27	3	160	1830	132
Spicy Buffalo Chicken Melt	14 oz.	880	47	13	4	98	2623	96

Items, Salads & Soups continued

	Serving	Calories	Total fat (gm)	Saturated fat (gm)	Trans fats (gm)	Cholesterol (mg)	Sodium (mg)	Carbs (gm)
Vegetable Beef	8 oz.	79	1	1	0	5	820	18
Chicken Noodle	8 oz.	110	6	1	1.5	25	1130	15
Broccoli & Cheddar	8 oz.	190	14	5	4	30	1020	15
Fish item	12 oz.	589	30	5	4	30	1557	30
Clam Chowder	8 oz.	624	42	34	3.5	5	1474	55
Taco Salad	16 oz.	505	22	11	NA	54	553	NA
Chef's Salad	17 oz.	365	16	7	0	289	1376	17
Grilled Chicken Breast Salad	13 oz.	259	11	5	0	90	724	10
Turkey Breast Salad w/o dressing	13 oz.	248	8	4	0	86	798	12
Fried Chicken Strip Salad	15 oz.	438	26	6	0	78	1030	26
Coleslaw	5 oz.	274	24	30	2.5	37	588	14
Side Caesar w/ dressing	6 oz.	362	26	7	0	23	913	20
Side Garden Salad w/o dressing	7 oz.	113	7	5	0	0	144	6
French Fries, unsalted	5 oz.	423	20	5	3	0	221	57
Seasoned Fries	4 oz.	261	12	3	4	0	556	35
Onion Rings	4 oz.	381	23	6	NA	6	1003	38

Appetizers & Entrées

	Serving	Calories	Total fat (gm)	Saturated fat (gm)	Trans fats (gm)	Cholesterol (mg)	Sodium (mg)	Carbs (gm)
Sampler	17 oz.	1405	80	24	1	75	5305	124
Buffalo Wings	9 items	974	72	18	0	267	4049	11
Mozzarella Sticks	8 items	710	41	24	0	48	5220	49
Smothered Cheese Fries	9 oz.	767	48	17	3	78	875	69
Buffalo Chicken Strips	5 items	734	42	4	0	96	1673	43
Chicken Strips	5 items	720	33	4	0	95	1666	56
Meat Loaf	1 item	930	60	25	0	145	4400	51
Mushroom Swiss Chopped Steak	1 item	800	73	29	0	173	1140	11
T-Bone Steak Dinner	14 oz.	860	65	29	0	196	867	0
Steakhouse Strip Dinner	8 oz.	410	27	18	0	136	635	NA
Country Fried Steak	9 oz.	644	46	10	0	89	2149	30
Steakhouse Strip & Shrimp	10 oz.	517	33	19	0	216	789	NA
Blackened Steakhouse Strip	10 oz.	775	66	25	0	136	1427	NA
Fried Shrimp Dinner	5 oz.	258	11	2	0	159	849	18
Roast Turkey & Stuffing w/ gravy	12 oz.	435	10	2	1	100	4620	66
Grilled Tilapia Dinner	11 oz.	470	18	5	0	201	1268	33
Lemon Pepper Tilapia	15 oz.	773	47	11	0	248	2852	38
Grilled Chicken Dinner	6 oz.	200	5	1	0	67	824	4
Grilled Chicken Alfredo	1 item	1290	67	29	1	235	1980	111
Hickory Grilled Chicken	15 oz.	766	48	16	0	186	6030	NA
Fish & Chips	17 oz.	958	54	30	0	88	1390	83
Chicken Strips	10 oz.	635	25	1	0	95	1510	55

Denny's® Continued

Appetizers & Entrées continued

	Serving	Calories	Total fat (gm)	Saturated fat (gm)	Trans fats (gm)	Cholesterol (mg)	Sodium (mg)	Carbs (gm)
Corn	4 oz.	110	2	0	0	0	180	23
Green Beans	4 oz.	40	1	0	0	0	47	NA
Baked Potato, plain w/ skin	7 oz.	220	0	0	0	0	16	51
Mashed Potatoes, plain	5 oz.	168	7	3	0	8	498	23
Vegetable Rice Pilaf	5 oz.	173	3	1	0	0	1033	33
Bread Stuffing, plain	3 oz.	100	1	0	NA	0	405	19
Cottage Cheese	3 oz.	72	3	2	NA	10	281	2
Musselman's Applesauce	3 oz.	60	0	0	0	0	13	15
Sliced Tomatoes (3 slices)	2 oz.	13	0	0	0	0	6	3

Desserts

	Serving	Calories	Total fat (gm)	Saturated fat (gm)	Trans fats (gm)	Cholesterol (mg)	Sodium (mg)	Carbs (gm)
Apple Pie	7 oz.	470	21	5	2	0	650	68
Coconut Cream Pie	7 oz.	701	32	20	1	1	963	100
French Silk Pie	7 oz.	737	56	31	0	96	353	58
Apple Crisp a la mode	12 oz.	723	21	8	0	32	394	133
Chocolate Peanut Butter Pie	6 oz.	653	39	19	2	27	319	64
Cheesecake	7 oz.	580	38	24	2	174	380	51
Carrot Cake	8 oz.	799	45	13	3	125	630	99
Hershey's Chocolate Cake	5 oz.	631	33	13	2	40	420	79
Hot Fudge Brownie a la Mode	10 oz.	997	42	6	3.5	14	82	147
Hot Fudge Brownie (kid's)	3 oz.	344	16	4	1.5	25	245	49
Banana Split	19 oz.	894	43	19	0	78	177	121
Double Scoop Sundae	6 oz.	375	27	12	0	74	86	29
Single Scoop Sundae (delicious dip)	3 oz.	188	14	6	0	37	43	14
Milkshake (vanilla/chocolate)	12 oz.	560	26	16	0	100	272	76
Malted Milkshake (vanilla/chocolate)	12 oz.	583	26	16	0	100	278	82
Floats (Root Beer or Cola)	12 oz.	280	10	6	0	39	109	47
Oreo Blender Blaster	15 oz.	895	46	23	0	135	280	112
Oreo Blender Blaster (kid's)	10 oz.	580	29	15	0	87	194	72

Kid's D-Zone

	Serving	Calories	Total fat (gm)	Saturated fat (gm)	Trans fats (gm)	Cholesterol (mg)	Sodium (mg)	Carbs (gm)
Alien Hotcakes w/ meat	6 oz.	463	22	7	NA	38	1410	49
Alien Hotcakes w/o meat	4 oz.	344	9	3	NA	13	1014	47
Junior Grand Slam	5 oz.	397	25	7	NA	230	1118	38
Big Dipper French Toastix	7 oz.	627	71	13	NA	190	1068	71
Little Dippers w/ marinara & fries	12 oz.	860	43	17	NA	22	1679	80
Little Dippers w/ applesauce & marinara	10 oz.	566	27	13	NA	22	1504	50
Burgerlicious	4 oz.	296	17	6	NA	28	368	NA
Cosmic Cheeseburger	4 oz.	341	20	6	NA	40	580	24

Denny's® Continued

Kid's D-Zone continued

	Serving	Calories	Total fat (gm)	Saturated fat (gm)	Trans fats (gm)	Cholesterol (mg)	Sodium (mg)	Carbs (gm)
Flying Saucer Pizza	4 oz.	331	14	5	0	16	514	38
Galactic Grilled Cheese	3 oz.	334	20	2	NA	24	828	28
Moon & Stars Chicken Nuggets	2 oz.	190	13	4	NA	30	340	9
Macaroni & Cheese	7 oz.	353	13	4	0	19	651	48
Thanksgiving Jr.	7 oz.	290	14	4	NA	27	3881	NA
Thanksgiving Jr. w/ red grapes	10 oz.	350	14	4	NA	27	3883	NA
Moon Crater Mashed Potatoes w/ brown gravy	5 oz.	145	6	2	NA	6	557	20
Cucumber Craverz	3 oz.	164	16	3	NA	14	232	NA
Astronaut Applesauce	3 oz.	84	0	0	NA	0	38	19
Goldfish Galaxy	2 oz.	284	3	9	NA	473	36	0
Deep-Sea Salad w/ ranch dressing	4 oz.	240	20	3	NA	16	359	13
Anti-Gravity Grapes	3 oz.	60	0	0	NA	0	2	15
Neutron Brownie (Kid's size)	3 oz.	344	16	4	NA	25	245	49
Delicious Dip Sundae	5 oz.	413	19	9	NA	44	111	59

Seniors Menu

	Serving	Calories	Total fat (gm)	Saturated fat (gm)	Trans fats (gm)	Cholesterol (mg)	Sodium (mg)	Carbs (gm)
Omelette	9 oz.	429	20	12	0.5	515	755	36
Scrambled Egg & Cheddar	12 oz.	735	51	17	0	553	2168	56
Starter	8 oz.	544	42	11	0	245	631	23
French Toast Slam	7 oz.	591	43	15	0	378	690	37
Belgian Waffle Slam	10 oz.	700	51	24	0	518	1764	29
Biscuits & Gravy	14 oz.	791	55	18	0	546	1488	NA
Grilled Tilapia	6 oz.	248	10	3	0	201	180	0
Lemon Pepper Tilapia	9 oz.	509	41	9	0	104	1821	6
Fried Shrimp Dinner	3.5 oz.	149	6	1	0	80	694	14
Pot Roast with Vegetable Blend	1 item	180	89	3	0	35	50	8
Turkey & Stuffing	10 oz.	360	9	2	1	69	4280	57
Grilled Chicken Breast	6 oz.	200	5	1	0	67	824	15
Country Fried Steak	5 oz.	341	23	5	0	44	1464	18
Chicken Strip Dinner	5 oz.	285	10	0	0	37	969	31
Club	9 oz.	540	31	5	0	89	1499	40
Bacon Cheddar Burger	7 oz.	433	25	8	0	57	608	27
Grilled Cheese Sandwich	7 oz.	510	30	14	0	54	1360	50
Fish & Chips	13 oz.	756	47	35	0	67	1116	64

Domino's® Pizza

12" Classic Hand-Tossed (1 of 8 Slices)

	Serving	Calories	Total fat (gm)	Saturated fat (gm)	Trans fats (gr)	Cholesterol (mg)	Sodium (mg)	Carbs (gm)
Beef	1 slice	225	9	4	0	16	493	30
Cheese	1 slice	186	6	2	0	9	385	29
Green Pepper, Onion, & Mushroom	1 slice	191	6	2	0	9	386	31
Ham	1 slice	198	6	3	0	13	492	30
Ham & Pineapple	1 slice	200	6	3	0	12	467	32
Pepperoni	1 slice	223	9	4	0	16	522	31
Pepperoni & Sausage	1 slice	255	12	5	0	22	626	32
Sausage	1 slice	231	10	4	0	17	530	31
America's Favorite Feast	1 slice	257	12	5	0	22	626	34
Bacon Cheeseburger Feast	1 slice	273	13	6	0	27	634	33
Barbecue Feast	1 slice	252	10	5	0	20	600	38
Deluxe Feast	1 slice	234	10	4	0	17	542	34
ExtravaganZZa Feast	1 slice	289	14	6	0	28	764	35
Hawaiian Feast	1 slice	223	8	4	0	16	547	35
MeatZZa Feast	1 slice	281	14	6	0	28	740	34
Pepperoni Feast	1 slice	265	13	5	0	24	670	34
Vegi Feast	1 slice	218	8	4	0	13	489	34

12" Crunchy Thin Crust

	Serving	Calories	Total fat (gm)	Saturated fat (gm)	Trans fats (gr)	Cholesterol (mg)	Sodium (mg)	Carbs (gm)
Beef	1 slice	175	11	4	0	17	400	14
Cheese	1 slice	137	7	3	0	10	293	15
Green Pepper, Onion, & Mushroom	1 slice	142	8	3	0	10	293	15
Ham	1 slice	148	8	3	0	14	400	14
Ham & Pineapple	1 slice	150	8	3	0	13	374	16
Pepperoni	1 slice	174	11	4	0	17	429	14
Pepperoni & Sausage	1 slice	206	14	5	0	23	533	15
Sausage	1 slice	181	11	4	0	18	438	15

12" Ultimate Deep Dish

	Serving	Calories	Total fat (gm)	Saturated fat (gm)	Trans fats (gr)	Cholesterol (mg)	Sodium (mg)	Carbs (gm)
Beef	1 slice	277	15	5	0	19	664	26
Cheese	1 slice	238	11	4	0	11	556	27
Green Pepper, Onion & Mushroom	1 slice	244	11	4	0	11	556	27
Ham	1 slice	250	12	4	0	16	663	26
Ham & Pineapple	1 slice	252	12	4	0	15	637	28
Pepperoni	1 slice	275	14	5	0	19	692	27
Pepperoni & Sausage	1 slice	307	17	6	0	25	796	26
Sausage	1 slice	283	15	5	0	19	701	27

Sides

	Serving	Calories	Total fat (gm)	Saturated fat (gm)	Trans fats (gr)	Cholesterol (mg)	Sodium (mg)	Carbs (gm)
Buffalo Chicken Kickers	1 item	47	2	1	0	9	163	27
Barbeque Buffalo Wings	1 item	50	3	1	0	26	176	6

Domino's® Pizza
Continued

Sides continued

	Serving	Calories	Total fat (gm)	Saturated fat (gm)	Trans fats (gm)	Cholesterol (mg)	Sodium (mg)	Carbs (gm)
Brownie Squares	1 item	160	7	2	0	15	95	NA
Hot Buffalo Wings	1 item	45	3	1	0	26	255	5
Breadsticks	1 item	115	6	1	0	0	122	14
Cheesy Bread	1 item	123	7	2	0	6	162	14
Cinna Stix	1 item	123	6	1	0	0	111	17
Salads								
Garden Fresh Salad	1 salad	70	4	2	0	10	85	5
Grilled Chicken Caesar Salad	1 salad	105	4	2	0	25	320	6

Don Pablo's®

Appetizers

	Serving	Calories	Total fat (gm)	Saturated fat (gm)	Trans fats (gm)	Cholesterol (mg)	Sodium (mg)	Carbs (gm)
Beef Taquitos	6 items	561	34	15	NA	73	1406	36
Chicken Flautas	6 items	507	31	12	NA	73	1505	39
Buffalo Wings	8 items	1036	78	16	NA	127	2326	NA
Chicken Nachos	1 order	1395	87	43	NA	254	2625	73
Cheese Nachos	1 order	1317	98	53	NA	231	1960	48
Steak Nachos	1 order	1430	99	48	NA	228	2480	71
Taco Beef Nachos	1 order	1625	113	55	NA	242	3308	85
The Don's Sampler	1 order	2002	118	55	NA	300	4074	129
Mesquite-Grilled Chicken Quesadilla	4 slices	665	32	16	NA	99	1348	55
Mesquite-Grilled Steak Quesadilla	4 slices	780	45	22	NA	94	1690	61
Cheese Quesadilla	4 slices	812	50	27	NA	115	1382	52
Portobella Mushroom & Vegetable Quesadilla	4 slices	752	42	17	NA	62	1465	NA
Smoked BBQ Chicken Quesadilla	4 slices	681	35	16	NA	77	1358	NA
Club Quesadilla	4 slices	872	50	23	NA	132	1870	NA
Fajitas								
Classic Chicken Fajitas	1 order	851	29	6	NA	121	2002	90
Classic Steak Fajitas	1 order	1174	68	24	NA	99	3074	106
Mesquite-Fired Chicken Fajitas	1 order	988	43	8	NA	121	2034	NA
Mesquite-Fired Black Angus Sirloin Fajitas	1 order	1185	55	13	NA	180	2324	NA
Mesquite-Fired Shrimp Fajitas	1 order	916	41	7	NA	308	1940	NA
Low Carb Black Angus Fajitas	1 order	680	45	24	NA	190	470	NA
Low Carb Smoked Chicken Fajitas	1 order	490	29	17	NA	130	1870	NA
Low Carb Mahi Mahi Fajitas	1 order	550	30	18	NA	225	570	NA

Don Pablo's®
Continued

Traditional Favorites

	Serving	Calories	Total fat (gm)	Saturated fat (gm)	Trans fats (gm)	Cholesterol (mg)	Sodium (mg)	Carbs (gm)
Real Burrito–Chicken	1 item	1099	42	20	NA	151	3255	NA
Real Burrito–Steak	1 item	1349	68	32	NA	141	4102	NA
Beef & Bean Burrito	1 item	1389	73	30	NA	154	3261	123
Beef Relleno	1 item	300	17	6	NA	37	1040	20
Cheese Relleno	1 item	400	26	14	NA	61	1100	19
Chicken Burrito	1 item	828	36	16	NA	117	3051	21
Chicken Chimichanga	1 item	1090	49	16	NA	95	3314	114
Chicken Relleno	1 item	235	11	3	NA	27	1120	21
Chicken Tamales	1 item	225	10	3	NA	19	600	25
Pork Tamales	1 item	270	14	5	NA	31	620	24
Spicy Ground Beef Chimi de Oro	1 item	1189	63	20	NA	107	2512	131
Traditional Pork Carnitas	1 item	1050	38	11	NA	118	3195	118

Tacos & Enchiladas

	Serving	Calories	Total fat (gm)	Saturated fat (gm)	Trans fats (gm)	Cholesterol (mg)	Sodium (mg)	Carbs (gm)
Crispy Beef Taco	1 taco	291	18	6	NA	36	350	36
Mama's Skinny Enchiladas	3 enchiladas	370	14	5	NA	73	2030	18
Soft Beef Taco	1 taco	327	18	7	NA	36	516	36
Spinach & Poblano Enchilada	1 enchilada	258	13	5	NA	9	1015	9
Three Amigos Enchiladas	3 enchiladas	700	16	21	NA	121	1990	18
Crispy Chicken Taco	1 taco	259	14	4	NA	35	520	34
Soft Chicken Taco	1 taco	295	13	5	NA	35	686	34
Cheese Enchilada	1 item	232	16	9	NA	39	565	39
Chicken Enchilada	1 item	213	13	5	NA	36	803	35
Beef Enchilada	1 item	263	18	7	NA	46	596	46

Little Amigos Menu

	Serving	Calories	Total fat (gm)	Saturated fat (gm)	Trans fats (gm)	Cholesterol (mg)	Sodium (mg)	Carbs (gm)
Fried Shrimp w/ tater tots	1 meal	528	24	8	NA	84	1325	NA
Cheese Enchilada w/ rice & Beans	1 meal	515	29	15	NA	66	1584	33
Beef Taco w/ rice & beans	1 meal	483	24	8	NA	43	983	50
Kid's Nachos-Original Queso	1 meal	478	30	11	NA	54	1309	NA
Grilled Cheese Crisp w/ tater tots	1 meal	883	48	21	NA	54	2363	92
Corn Dog w/ tater tots	1 meal	724	40	10	NA	30	2598	80
Chicken Stix w/ tater tots	1 meal	739	46	11	NA	33	1911	75

Side Items

	Serving	Calories	Total fat (gm)	Saturated fat (gm)	Trans fats (gm)	Cholesterol (mg)	Sodium (mg)	Carbs (gm)
Sweet Corn Cake	4 oz.	250	12	2	NA	0	556	NA
Mexican Rice	3 oz.	107	1	0	NA	0	416	21
Refritos	5 oz.	181	6	2	NA	0	551	31
Black Beans	4 oz.	119	2	0	NA	3	383	20
Charra Beans	5 oz.	96	2	0	NA	0	333	16
Chili Mashed Potatoes	2.75 oz.	108	6	2	NA	2	373	12

Don Pablo's®
Continued

Side Items continued	Serving	Calories	Total fat (gm)	Saturated fat (gm)	Trans fats (gm)	Cholesterol (mg)	Sodium (mg)	Carbs (gm)
Flour Tortilla Taco Shell	1 shell	490	27	5	NA	0	430	NA
Garden Vegetables	6 oz.	98	5	1	NA	0	305	13
Saffron Rice	3 oz.	140	6	5	NA	15	30	NA
White Chicken Chili-cup	6 oz.	234	13	3	NA	43	830	23
Salad								
Caesar Salad	1 salad	1390	114	18	NA	54	1580	79
Caesar Salad w/ Chicken	1 salad	1565	118	20	NA	54	2200	85
Caesar Salad w/ Steak	1 salad	1795	44	31	NA	119	2890	97
Tortilla Salad	1 salad	550	29	7	NA	14	434	59

Fast Food Factoid:

Dunkin' Donuts has the honor of being one of two fast food restaurants that has all or most of its foods coded red. Can you guess which other restaurant shares this distinction?
Krispy Kreme.

NOTES:

_____

_____

_____

_____

_____

_____

_____

_____

_____

Dunkin' Donuts®

	Serving	Calories	Total fat (gm)	Saturated fat (gm)	Trans fats (gm)	Cholesterol (mg)	Sodium (mg)	Carbs (gm)
Yeast Donuts								
Glazed	1 item	230	10	4.5	0	0	250	30
Apple Crumb	1 item	320	13	6	0	0	270	46
Blueberry Crumb	1 item	330	13	6	0	0	260	48
Chocolate Frosted	1 item	230	11	4.5	0	0	260	29
Jelly-Filled	1 item	270	10	4.5	0	0	280	39
Maple Frosted	1 item	240	10	4.5	0	0	260	31
Marble Frosted	1 item	230	11	4.5	0	0	260	30
Sugar Raised	1 item	210	10	4.5	0	0	250	27
French Crueller	1 item	150	8	5	0	20	105	17
Kreme Filled Donuts								
Bavarian Kreme	1 item	250	11	4.5	0	0	270	35
Boston Kreme	1 item	270	12	5	0	0	280	38
Chocolate Kreme	1 item	300	14	6	0	0	260	39
Vanilla Kreme	1 item	320	16	7	0	0	250	39
Cake Donuts								
Old-Fashioned	1 item	280	18	9	0	25	330	26
Glazed	1 item	330	18	9	0	25	340	38
Apple Crumb	1 item	290	15	3	1	15	320	NA
Blueberry	1 item	290	16	6	0	10	400	35
Chocolate Frosted	1 item	330	19	9	0	25	350	36
Frosted Lemon	1 item	240	14	4	3	0	150	NA
Powdered	1 item	310	18	9	0	25	330	34
Whole Wheat Glazed	1 item	310	19	8	0	0	380	32
Stick Donuts								
Plain Cake	1 item	310	20	10	0	35	310	29
Glazed Cake	1 item	360	20	10	0	35	310	41
Powdered Cake	1 item	340	20	10	0	35	310	37
Jelly Filled	1 item	420	20	10	0	35	320	53
Fancies & Munchkins								
Glazed Fritter	1 item	250	13	6	0	0	330	31
Apple Fritter	1 item	290	13	6	0	0	360	35
Chocolate-Iced Bismark	1 item	340	15	6	0	0	290	50
Bow Tie	1 item	300	17	8	0	0	340	34
Éclair	1 item	300	15	6	0	0	290	39
Plain Cake Munchkins	4 items	230	15	7	0	25	240	21
Glazed Cake Munchkins	4 items	300	15	7	0	20	190	38
Powdered Cake Munchkins	4 items	260	15	7	0	25	210	29

Einstein Bros. Bagels®

Bagels

	Serving	Calories	Total fat (gm)	Saturated fat (gm)	Trans fats (gm)	Cholesterol (mg)	Sodium (mg)	Carbs (gm)
Plain	1 item	320	1	0	0	0	520	62
Asiago Cheese	1 item	360	3	2	0	5	570	71
Chocolate Chip	1 item	340	3	2	0	0	520	68
Chopped Garlic	1 item	380	3	1	0	0	680	79
Chopped Onion	1 item	330	1	0	0	0	500	71
Cinnamon Raisin Swirl	1 item	320	2	0	0	70	510	70
Cinnamon Sugar	1 item	420	16	10	0	69	690	69
Cranberry	1 item	350	1	0	0	0	490	70
Egg	1 item	340	3	1	0	35	510	69
Everything	1 item	340	2	0	0	0	820	75
Honey Wheat	1 item	320	1	0	0	0	470	64
Jalapeno	1 item	290	3	2	0	0	520	61
Marble Rye	1 item	340	2	0	0	0	690	73
Nutty Banana	1 item	360	3	1	0	0	510	NA
Poppy Dip	1 item	350	2	0	0	0	680	74
Dark Pumpernickel	1 item	320	1	0	0	0	730	68
Potato	1 item	230	5	1	0	0	600	62
Pumpkin	1 item	310	2	0	0	0	590	61
Sun-Dried Tomato	1 item	320	1	0	0	0	520	60
Wild Blueberry	1 item	350	1	0	0	0	510	70
Lower Carb 9-Grain	1 item	210	4	1	0	0	650	NA
9-Grain Plain w/ cream cheese	1 item	310	13	7	0	30	730	NA

Cream Cheese Shmear (whipped)

	Serving	Calories	Total fat (gm)	Saturated fat (gm)	Trans fats (gm)	Cholesterol (mg)	Sodium (mg)	Carbs (gm)
Plain	2 Tbsp	70	7	5	0	20	65	1
Plain (reduced-fat)	2 Tbsp	60	5	4	0	15	85	2
Blueberry	2 Tbsp	70	5	4	0	15	50	6
Garden Vegetable	2 Tbsp	60	5	4	0	15	100	3
Honey Almond (reduced-fat)	2 Tbsp	70	5	3	0	15	45	6
Onion & Chive	2 Tbsp	70	6	4	0	20	60	3
Strawberry	2 Tbsp	70	5	4	0	15	50	5

Specialty Teas & Coffees

	Serving	Calories	Total fat (gm)	Saturated fat (gm)	Trans fats (gm)	Cholesterol (mg)	Sodium (mg)	Carbs (gm)
Americano Regular	8 fl. oz.	1	0	0	0	0	0	0
Specialty Hot Tea	8 fl. oz.	0	0	0	0	0	0	0
Coffee (regular decaf)	12 fl. oz.	0	0	0	0	0	0	0
Café Latte	12 fl. oz.	140	5	4	0	20	140	13
Non-Fat Café Latte	12 fl. oz.	100	1	0	0	5	150	14
Cappuccino	12 fl. oz.	90	4	2	0	15	95	9
Non-Fat Cappuccino	12 fl. oz.	60	0	0	0	5	95	9
Espresso	1.5 fl oz	1	0	0	0	0	0	0

Einstein Bros. Bagels® Continued

	Serving	Calories	Total fat (gm)	Saturated fat (gm)	Trans fats (gm)	Cholesterol (mg)	Sodium (mg)	Carbs (gm)
Specialty Teas & Coffees continued								
Mocha	12 fl oz	310	16	9	0	60	135	34
Low-Fat Mocha	12 fl oz	240	10	6	0	40	135	29
Deli Items								
Albacore Tuna on Artisan Wheat	1 item	400	9	1	0	35	520	48
Black Forest Ham on Challah	1 item	570	23	8	0	80	2000	NA
Chicken Caesar on Onion Challah	1 item	750	42	13	0	105	1450	61
Calypso Chicken Salad Sandwich	1 item	460	9	1	0	40	1100	NA
Club Mex on Challah	1 item	620	28	10	0	95	1820	59
Cobbie on Challah	1 item	610	28	10	0	80	1780	NA
Einstein Club on Rustic White	1 item	660	26	6	0	85	1350	NA
Grilled Chicken Bacon & Swiss	1 item	800	50	12	0	120	1410	49
Roasted Turkey on Artisan Wheat	1 item	600	28	9	0	95	1240	NA
Spicy Chicken on Onion Challah	1 item	540	22	7	0	85	1710	59
Stacked Roast Beef on Challah	1 item	540	24	10	0	80	2070	53
Tasty Turkey on Asiago Bagel	1 item	610	18	11	0	90	1490	81
Thai Chicken Sandwich w/ Peanut Poppyseed	1 item	560	22	4	0	60	1990	60
Veg Out on Sesame Seed	1 item	500	13	7	0	30	690	82
Bagel Dogs								
Andouille Sausage Onion Bagel Dog	1 item	540	20	8	0	60	1330	67
Chicago Bagel Dog on Asiago Bagel	1 item	740	35	15	0	80	1360	NA
Chicago Bagel Dog on Onion Bagel w/o cheese	1 item	680	30	12	0	70	1220	NA
Chicago Chili Cheese Bagel Dog	1 item	810	38	17	0	105	1550	NA
Chicken Portabello Sesame Bagel Dog	1 item	480	12	3	0	85	1240	68
Polish Sausage & Everything Bagel Dog	1 item	580	24	9	0	60	1680	66
Lower Carb 9-Grain Bagel Items								
Bagel Dog	1 item	560	33	13	0	70	1370	NA
Turkey Deli	1 item	330	6	2	0	45	1550	NA
Tuna Salad	1 item	360	9	2	0	35	1170	NA
Tasty Turkey	1 item	490	19	10	0	90	1550	NA
Frittata Egg	1 item	470	22	10	0	415	970	NA
Frittata Egg & Bacon	1 item	570	29	13	0	440	1230	NA
Frittata Egg w/ turkey sausage	1 item	550	26	11	0	445	1300	NA
Frittata Egg w/ Black Forest ham	1 item	550	24	11	0	445	1560	NA
Panini Items								
Albacore Panini Tuna Melt	1 item	530	21	7	0	60	1670	51

Einstein Bros. Bagels® Continued

Panini Items continued

	Serving	Calories	Total fat (gm)	Saturated fat (gm)	Trans fats (gm)	Cholesterol (mg)	Sodium (mg)	Carbs (gm)
Cali Club	1 item	750	34	11	NA	95	2120	NA
Cheesesteak Panini	1 item	735	33	11	0	85	2450	73
Ham & Cheese	1 item	620	22	10	NA	90	1930	65
Italian Chicken	1 item	690	27	10	NA	95	1460	68
Turkey Club Panini	1 item	840	41	12	0	110	2440	71

El Pollo Loco®

Flame-Grilled Chicken

	Serving	Calories	Total fat (gm)	Saturated fat (gm)	Trans fats (gm)	Cholesterol (mg)	Sodium (mg)	Carbs (gm)
Chicken Breast	1 item	187	7	2	0	128	540	0
Chicken Breast w/ skin removed	1 item	153	4	1	0	95	540	0
Leg	1 item	86	3	0	0	80	206	0
Thigh	1 item	120	7	2	0	82	225	0
Wing	1 item	83	3	1	0	58	334	0

Burritos

	Serving	Calories	Total fat (gm)	Saturated fat (gm)	Trans fats (gm)	Cholesterol (mg)	Sodium (mg)	Carbs (gm)
Twiced-Grilled Burrito	1 item	853	41	17	0	151	2936	58
Grilled Fiesta Burrito	1 item	1068	54	13	0	124	3006	0
Ultimate Chicken Burrito	1 item	701	24	8	0	65	2281	80
BRC Burrito	1 item	528	15	5	0	15	1394	61
BBQ Black Bean BRC Burrito	1 item	420	11	4	0	15	965	NA
BBQ Black Bean Classic Burrito	1 item	530	16	6	0	95	1315	NA
Classic Chicken Burrito	1 item	636	19	6	0	63	1749	63
Spicy Chicken Burrito	1 item	555	19	6	0	72	1962	NA
Chicken Lover's Burrito	1 item	526	18	6	0	101	1808	NA
Pollo Asado Burrito	1 item	599	23	6	0	156	2110	58

Pollo Salads

	Serving	Calories	Total fat (gm)	Saturated fat (gm)	Trans fats (gm)	Cholesterol (mg)	Sodium (mg)	Carbs (gm)
Tostado Salad	1 salad	740	33	9	0	65	1823	76
Tostado Salad w/o shell	1 salad	414	16	6	0	65	1479	42
Caesar Pollo Salad w/ dressing	1 salad	535	42	7	0	59	1242	17
Caesar Pollo Salad w/o dressing	1 salad	221	9	2	0	44	908	15
Fiesta Pollo Salad w/ dressing	1 salad	747	57	15	0	97	1654	NA
Fiesta Pollo Salad w/o dressing	1 salad	439	26	11	0	82	1249	NA
Loco Salad w/ Creamy Cilantro Dressing	1 salad	179	14	3	0	10	210	7
Monterey Pollo Salad w/ dressing	1 salad	258	13	3	0	52	1266	NA
Monterey Pollo Salad w/o dressing	1 salad	176	6	1	0	44	836	NA

Bowls & Loco Favorites

	Serving	Calories	Total fat (gm)	Saturated fat (gm)	Trans fats (gm)	Cholesterol (mg)	Sodium (mg)	Carbs (gm)
Pollo Bowl w/o dressing	1 salad	543	10	1	0	42	2159	85
BBQ Chicken Quesadilla	1 item	670	31	15	0	140	1670	NA

El Pollo Loco®
Continued

Bowls & Loco Favorites continued

	Serving	Calories	Total fat (gm)	Saturated fat (gm)	Trans fats (gm)	Cholesterol (mg)	Sodium (mg)	Carbs (gm)
Chicken Caesar Bowl w/o dressing	1 salad	535	29	6	0	51	1451	45
Chicken Nachos	17.5 oz.	1299	77	31	0	202	2340	99
Chicken Tortilla Soup	1 item	210	9	3	0	60	1050	18
Chicken Quesadilla	1 item	654	30	15	0	108	1530	53
Cheese Quesadilla	1 item	543	26	14	0	60	1177	35
Chicken Taquitos	2 items	370	17	4	0	25	690	18
Chicken Soft Taco	1 taco	237	11	5	0	45	526	19
Taco al Carbon	1 taco	134	3	1	0	29	224	17

Kid's Meals

	Serving	Calories	Total fat (gm)	Saturated fat (gm)	Trans fats (gm)	Cholesterol (mg)	Sodium (mg)	Carbs (gm)
Popcorn Chicken	4 oz.	226	12	2	0	53	787	10
Cheese Quesadilla	1 item	420	23	13	0	60	610	35
Chicken Drumstick	1 item	86	3	0	0	80	206	0
French Fries	3 oz.	242	10	3	0	0	330	31

Side Dishes

	Serving	Calories	Total fat (gm)	Saturated fat (gm)	Trans fats (gm)	Cholesterol (mg)	Sodium (mg)	Carbs (gm)
Black Beans	6 oz.	306	16	6	0	13	731	NA
Cole Slaw	5 oz.	206	16	3	0	11	358	8
Corn Cobbette	1 item	42	0	0	0	0	7	19
French Fries	5.5 oz.	444	19	5	0	0	605	57
Garden Salad w/o dressing	1 salad	111	7	3	0	15	271	9
Macaroni & Cheese	5 .5 oz.	381	26	16	0	65	891	28
Mashed Potatoes	5 oz.	110	1	0	0	0	406	20
Gravy	1 oz.	12	0	0	0	1	151	2
Pinto Beans	6 oz.	154	4	0	0	0	674	25
Refried Beans w/ Cheese	1 item	270	7	2	0	10	730	36
Spanish Rice	4 oz.	161	1	0	0	0	421	64
Vegetables	4 oz.	68	4	1	0	0	78	8

Fazoli's®

Classic Pastas

	Serving	Calories	Total fat (gm)	Saturated fat (gm)	Trans fats (gm)	Cholesterol (mg)	Sodium (mg)	Carbs (gm)
Spaghetti w/ marinara sauce	small	440	3	0	0	0	770	88
Spaghetti w/ meat sauce	small	460	4	2	0	5	900	87
Spaghetti w/ meatballs	small	690	20	8	0	55	1470	94
Fettuccine Alfredo	small	500	11	4	0	15	870	83
Fettuccine Alfredo w/ broccoli	small	590	17	5	0	15	1320	88
Peppery Chicken Alfredo	small	570	12	4	0	55	1190	84
Roasted Garlic Alfredo	1 order	710	17	5	0	60	2210	NA
Ravioli w/ marinara sauce	1 order	580	15	7	0	60	1350	71

Fazoli's® Continued

	Serving	Calories	Total fat (gm)	Saturated fat (gm)	Trans fats (gm)	Cholesterol (mg)	Sodium (mg)	Carbs (gm)
Classic Pastas continued								
Ravioli w/ meat sauce	1 order	610	16	8	0	65	1480	71
Six-Layer Lasagna	1 order	620	23	11	1	50	2020	NA
Six-Layer Lasagna w/ broccoli	1 order	680	28	12	1	55	2290	NA
Classic Sampler	1 order	790	18	8	0	35	1880	110
Ultimate Sampler	1 order	1010	29	13	1	60	2700	134
Classic Ziti w/ meat sauce	1 order	500	24	14	0	60	1820	65
Garden-Style Chicken Penne	1 order	770	24	4	0	40	2550	NA
Penne Marinara	1 order	430	2	0	0	0	750	88
Penne w/ meat sauce	1 order	460	4	1	0	5	880	87
Penne w/ meatballs	1 order	680	20	8	0	55	1450	93
Penne Marinara w/ black pepper chicken strips	1 order	520	5	1	0	35	1170	88
Roma Chicken Panini	1 order	740	36	9	0	100	1790	NA
Grilled Chicken Panini	1 order	420	7	3	0	65	2030	56
Oven-Baked								
Tuscan Chicken Bake	1 order	660	29	14	0	125	1800	NA
Baked Chicken Parmesan	1 order	760	16	4	0	65	1720	117
Twice Baked Lasagna	1 order	890	43	24	1	110	2770	NA
Baked Spaghetti	1 order	710	24	14	0	65	1290	90
Baked Spaghetti w/ meatballs	1 order	970	42	22	1	120	2010	100
Rigatoni Romano	1 order	1090	54	20	1	135	3180	101
Twice-Baked Ziti w/ meat sauce	1 order	1340	81	49	0	235	4250	65
Chicken Broccoli Bake	1 order	560	27	14	0	170	3590	76
9" Brick-Oven Style Pizza								
Ultimate Cheese	1 pizza	800	32	16	0	60	1970	31
Pepperoni	1 pizza	870	39	16	0	70	2410	31
Italian Meat	1 pizza	970	46	19	0	85	2880	NA
Mediterranean	1 pizza	890	43	17	0	90	2420	NA
Spicy Southwest Chicken	1 pizza	830	32	13	0	85	2340	NA
7" Submarino Sandwiches								
Original	1 item	1390	78	22	0	135	3320	68
Club	1 item	1040	44	12	0	105	2630	68
Ham & Swiss	1 item	980	38	10	0	95	2240	65
Italian Deli	1 item	840	18	7	0	75	3650	68
Meatball	1 item	1110	44	20	1	125	2750	NA
Turkey	1 item	940	36	9	0	80	2500	NA
7" Panini Sandwiches								
Four Cheese & Tomato	1 item	820	52	21	1	105	1290	53
Chicken Caesar Club	1 item	740	41	16	0	135	1730	NA

Fazoli's® Continued

	Serving	Calories	Total fat (gm)	Saturated fat (gm)	Trans fats (gm)	Cholesterol (mg)	Sodium (mg)	Carbs (gm)
7" Panini Sandwiches continued								
Chicken Pesto	1 item	580	28	8	0	65	1400	NA
Grilled Chicken	1 item	380	7	3	0	50	1360	56
Smoked Turkey	1 item	710	40	12	0	100	2110	54
Kid's Meals								
Spaghetti w/ marinara sauce	1 order	260	1	0	0	0	370	53
Spaghetti w/ meat sauce	1 order	270	2	0	0	0	440	53
Spaghetti w/ meatballs	1 order	340	7	3	0	20	610	55
Baked Ziti	1 order	270	13	7	0	35	970	25
Lasagna	1 order	310	11	5	0	25	1000	21
Cheese Ravioli w/ marinara sauce	1 order	290	7	4	3	660	43	43
Kid's Cheese Ravioli w/ meat sauce	1 order	300	8	4	0	30	730	42
Kid's Fettuccine Alfredo	1 order	290	5	2	0	5	420	50
Kid's Cheese Pizza	1 pizza	380	15	8	0	30	990	31
Kid's Pepperoni Pizza	1 pizza	450	21	10	0	45	1260	31
Salads								
Garden Side Salad w/o dressing	1 salad	25	0	0	0	0	30	4
Caesar Side Salad	1 salad	110	5	2	0	5	270	4
Pasta Side Salad	1 salad	240	14	4	0	15	1030	41
Chicken Caesar Salad	1 salad	190	6	2	0	45	520	NA
Chicken BLT Ranch	1 salad	270	10	4	0	80	1060	13
Chicken & Fruit	1 salad	270	2	0	0	55	700	28
Chicken & Pasta Caesar Salad	1 salad	520	34	7	0	90	1670	36
Grilled Chicken Salad w/o dressing	1 salad	110	2	0	0	40	370	NA
Italian Market Salad	1 salad	620	41	13	0	90	2910	NA
Breadstick	1 item	140	6	1	1	0	250	20
Dry Breadstick	1 item	100	2	0	0	0	150	20
Minestrone Soup	1 bowl	90	2	1	0	0	950	NA
Parmesan Chicken Salad	1 salad	360	15	5	0	65	850	NA
Herb Chicken Noodle Soup	1 bowl	70	1	0	0	15	200	NA
Tomato Florentine Soup	1 bowl	130	8	3	0	10	650	NA

Friendly's Ice Cream®
Does not provide nutrition information.

Godfather's Pizza®

	Serving	Calories	Total fat (gm)	Saturated fat (gm)	Trans fats (gm)	Cholesterol (mg)	Sodium (mg)	Carbs (gm)
Original Crust (medium)								
All Meat Combo	1 slice	373	16	NA	0	39	905	35
Bacon Cheeseburger	1 slice	328	13	NA	0	35	795	35
Cheese	1 slice	260	7	NA	0	15	455	34
Combo	1 slice	350	14	NA	0	30	850	37
Hawaiian	1 slice	281	8	NA	0	19	549	38
Hot Stuff	1 slice	360	6	NA	0	35	840	35
Humble Pie	1 slice	379	18	NA	0	37	752	35
Pepperoni	1 slice	294	10	NA	0	22	579	34
Taco	1 slice	362	16	NA	0	42	810	36
Veggie	1 slice	275	8	NA	0	15	524	36
Golden Crust (medium)								
All Meat Combo	1 slice	285	13	NA	0	27	654	27
Bacon Cheeseburger	1 slice	267	12	NA	0	27	620	26
Cheese	1 slice	221	8	NA	0	13	371	26
Combo	1 slice	290	13	NA	0	25	650	28
Hawaiian	1 slice	238	8	NA	0	16	464	29
Hot Stuff	1 slice	290	14	NA	0	25	620	27
Humble Pie	1 slice	306	15	NA	0	29	589	27
Pepperoni	1 slice	255	11	NA	0	19	495	26
Taco	1 slice	300	14	NA	0	35	619	27
Veggie	1 slice	232	8	NA	0	13	416	27
Thin Crust (medium)								
All Meat Combo	1 slice	282	15	NA	0	31	607	20
Bacon Cheeseburger	1 slice	246	13	NA	0	28	521	20
Cheese	1 slice	200	9	NA	0	14	271	16
Combo	1 slice	250	13	NA	0	25	540	18
Hawaiian	1 slice	217	9	NA	0	17	365	19
Hot Stuff	1 slice	270	15	NA	0	30	550	20
Humble Pie	1 slice	285	16	NA	0	30	490	17
Pepperoni	1 slice	234	12	NA	0	20	395	16
Taco	1 slice	278	15	NA	0	35	520	17
Veggie	1 slice	209	9	NA	0	14	317	18
Dessert Pizza (medium)								
Cinnamon Streusel	1 slice	228	6	NA	0	0	208	40
M&M Streusel	1 slice	263	7	NA	0	1	212	45
Monkey Bread	1/6 order	120	120	NA	0	0	130	23
Apple	1 slice	206	4	NA	0	0	204	39
Cherry	1 slice	210	4	NA	0	0	193	40

Godfather's Pizza® Continued

Side Items

	Serving	Calories	Total fat (gm)	Saturated fat (gm)	Trans fats (gm)	Cholesterol (mg)	Sodium (mg)	Carbs (gm)
Breadsticks	1 item	80	2	NA	0	0	71	14
Cheesesticks	1 item	132	4	NA	0	6	197	18
Potato Wedges	4 oz.	192	9	NA	3.7	0	342	24
Chocolate Chip Cookie	1 item	195	8	NA	0	21	157	30

Golden Corral®

Breakfast

	Serving	Calories	Total fat (gm)	Saturated fat (gm)	Trans fats (gm)	Cholesterol (mg)	Sodium (mg)	Carbs (gm)
Scrambled Eggs	3.5 oz.	160	11	4	NA	390	210	2
Corned Beef Hash	1 cup	420	30	13	NA	90	1590	22
Creamed Chipped Beef	½ cup	175	11	2	NA	15	570	9
Bacon	3 items	180	14	5	NA	30	540	1
Sausage Links	3 links	160	14	4	NA	35	460	1
Sausage Patties	1 item	247	21	7	NA	64	552	0
Split Smoked Sausage	1 item	250	23	10	NA	40	790	2
French Toast	1 slice	241	8	0	NA	0	329	23
Hash Browns	½ cup	102	7	0	NA	0	76	8
Hash Brown Casserole	½ cup	155	7	0	NA	0	520	17
Sausage Gravy	1 oz.	41	3	1	NA	4	124	2

Soups

	Serving	Calories	Total fat (gm)	Saturated fat (gm)	Trans fats (gm)	Cholesterol (mg)	Sodium (mg)	Carbs (gm)
Broccoli Cheese w/ florets	½ cup	160	9	5	NA	10	900	8
Chicken Gumbo	½ cup	70	2	0	NA	10	740	10
Chicken Noodle	½ cup	100	3	1	NA	55	1240	12
Timberline Chili	1 cup.	280	13	5	NA	30	1240	23
Clam Chowder	½ cup	140	6	2	NA	10	1110	17
Potato w/ bacon	½ cup	120	5	1	NA	5	980	17
Tomato Pasta Florentine	½ cup	90	2	1	NA	0	1080	NA
Vegetable Beef	½ cup	100	2	1	NA	5	1230	17

Salads

	Serving	Calories	Total fat (gm)	Saturated fat (gm)	Trans fats (gm)	Cholesterol (mg)	Sodium (mg)	Carbs (gm)
Carrot & Raisin Salad	½ cup	113	5	0	0	0	124	17
Macaroni Salad	½ cup	190	8	0	0	0	400	26
Marinated Mushroom Salad	½ cup	103	7	0	0	0	380	6
Marinated Vegetable Salad	½ cup	47	2	0	0	0	140	5
Tuna Salad	½ cup	237	12	0	0	0	532	8

Entrées

	Serving	Calories	Total fat (gm)	Saturated fat (gm)	Trans fats (gm)	Cholesterol (mg)	Sodium (mg)	Carbs (gm)
Asian Pork Roast	1 cup	510	34	10	NA	275	1500	10
BBQ Chicken (Leg Quarter)	1 items	480	22	8	NA	200	1080	20
BBQ Pork	3 oz.	170	8	3	NA	75	105	5

Golden Corral®
Continued
Entrées continued

	Serving	Calories	Total fat (gm)	Saturated fat (gm)	Trans fats (gm)	Cholesterol (mg)	Sodium (mg)	Carbs (gm)
Sirloin Steak	3 oz.	219	13	0	NA	0	983	0
Steakburgers	6 oz.	759	55	0	NA	0	1754	0
Pot Roast	3.5 oz.	206	12	5	NA	93	229	1
Roast Beef	3 oz.	183	10	0	NA	0	134	1
Meatloaf	3.5 oz.	190	10	4	NA	90	520	10
Ham	2 oz.	80	2	1	NA	30	560	1
Pork Chop	1 Chop	200	13	5	NA	65	400	0
Grilled Pork Chop or Loin Slices	3 oz.	119	4	0	NA	0	153	0
Roast Herb Pork Chop	3 oz.	334	17	0	NA	0	1619	6
Rotisserie Chicken (breast/wing)	6 oz.	320	15	5	NA	185	1100	0
Fried Chicken (leg/thigh)	3 oz.	250	19	9	NA	60	520	2
Bourbon Street Chicken	3.5 oz.	210	11	4	NA	115	410	5
Turkey Breast	2 oz.	70	3	1	NA	30	340	1
Carved Salmon	2 oz.	138	9	0	NA	0	274	0
Cajun Whitefish	3 oz.	110	7	0	NA	0	859	0
Cajun-Style Fish Fillet	2 items	210	9	0	NA	0	650	19
Cracker Crumb Fish Fillet	2 items	229	13	0	NA	3	480	17
Salmon Fillet	2 oz.	138	9	NA	NA	NA	274	0
Salmon Steaks w/ Lemon Herb Butter	3.5 oz.	208	14	NA	NA	NA	480	4

Pasta Side Items

	Serving	Calories	Total fat (gm)	Saturated fat (gm)	Trans fats (gm)	Cholesterol (mg)	Sodium (mg)	Carbs (gm)
Buttered Noodles	½ cup	163	4	0	NA	0	7	24
Creamy Chicken & Pasta	1 cup	210	6	3	NA	40	980	25
Macaroni & Beef	1 cup	260	11	5	NA	30	1260	26
Macaroni & Cheese	1 cup	400	18	8	NA	30	1010	42
Spaghetti Pasta	2 oz.	210	1	0	NA	0	0	42
Spaghetti Sauce	½ cup	110	0	0	NA	0	510	25
Lasagna w/ meat sauce	1 cup	290	11	6	NA	30	910	NA

Hot Side Items

	Serving	Calories	Total fat (gm)	Saturated fat (gm)	Trans fats (gm)	Cholesterol (mg)	Sodium (mg)	Carbs (gm)
Baked Potato (plain)	1 item	109	0	0	NA	0	8	25
Broccoli & Rice	½ cup	220	5	0	NA	0	520	36
Mashed Potatoes	3.5 oz.	120	6	2	NA	0	260	14
Brown Gravy	1 oz.	100	4	1	NA	2	1320	16
Chicken Gravy	1 oz.	104	4	1	NA	4	1366	NA
Sweet Potato	1 item	137	0	0	NA	0	17	32
White Rice	½ cup	178	5	0	NA	0	289	27

Vegetables

	Serving	Calories	Total fat (gm)	Saturated fat (gm)	Trans fats (gm)	Cholesterol (mg)	Sodium (mg)	Carbs (gm)
Escalloped Apples	2/3 cup	180	2	1	NA	0	20	40
Steamed Broccoli	½ cup	25	1	0	NA	0	170	5

Golden Corral®
Continued
Vegetables continued

	Serving	Calories	Total fat (gm)	Saturated fat (gm)	Trans fats (gm)	Cholesterol (mg)	Sodium (mg)	Carbs (gm)
Steamed Cabbage	½ cup	60	5	0	NA	0	80	1
Southern-Style Cabbage	½ cup	26	1	0	NA	0	95	4
Steamed Carrots	½ cup	79	5	0	NA	0	97	6
Steamed Cauliflower	½ cup	13	0	0	NA	0	162	2
Cheddar Cheese Sauce	¼ cup	110	9	4	NA	15	540	4
Corn	1 cup	310	9	0	NA	0	94	52
Corn on the Cob	1 item	106	2	0	NA	0	20	22
Green Beans	½ cup	34	0	0	NA	0	415	6
Green & Yellow Beans	½ cup	71	5	0	NA	0	76	4
Black Eyed Peas	½ cup	149	1	0	NA	0	500	28
Green Peas	½ cup	109	6	0	NA	0	78	10
Northern Beans	½ cup	149	1	0	NA	0	500	28
Pinto Beans	½ cup	149	1	0	NA	0	500	28
Spinach	½ cup	34	1	0	NA	0	172	2
Creamed Spinach	½ cup	180	13	5	NA	15	410	11
Squash Medley	½ cup	66	5	0	NA	0	79	3
Vegetable Trio	½ cup	25	0	0	NA	0	170	NA
Yams & Apples	½ cup	160	2	1	NA	0	110	35
Steamed Zucchini	½ cup	60	5	0	NA	0	76	1
Bakery Items								
Skillet Cornbread	3 oz.	85	2	0	NA	0	228	22
Corn Muffin	3 oz.	204	5	0	NA	0	549	32
Mexican Corn Muffin	3 oz.	96	3	0	NA	0	265	NA
Kaiser Roll	1 roll	160	1	1	NA	0	350	31
Yeast Roll w/o butter	1 roll	195	2	1	NA	0	344	42

Fast Food Factoid:

Exercise is like a combination of psychotherapy, physical therapy, and stress management all concentrated in one 30-minute session.

Dr. Steven Aldana, The Culprit and The Cure

NOTES:

_____

_____

_____

_____

Hardee's®

	Serving	Calories	Total fat (gm)	Saturated fat (gm)	Trans fats (gm)	Cholesterol (mg)	Sodium (mg)	Carbs (gm)
Breakfast								
Big Country Breakfast Platter w/ Breaded Pork Chops	1 meal	1220	68	13	NA	465	2230	102
Big Country Breakfast Platter w/ bacon	1 meal	980	56	13	NA	435	2080	90
Big Country Breakfast Platter w/ chicken	1 meal	1140	61	13	NA	480	2580	105
Big Country Breakfast Platter w/ country steak	1 meal	1150	68	16	NA	455	2660	98
Big Country Breakfast Platter w/ country ham	1 meal	970	53	12	NA	460	2600	90
Big Country Breakfast Platter w/ breakfast ham	1 meal	970	52	12	NA	455	2450	90
Big Country Breakfast Platter w/ sausage	1 meal	1060	64	15	NA	455	2140	91
Low Carb Breakfast Bowl	1 meal	620	50	21	NA	325	1380	6
Loaded Biscuit & Gravy Bowl	1 meal	770	54	15	NA	245	1950	49
Biscuit 'n Gravy	9 oz.	530	34	8	NA	10	1550	47
Pancakes	3 items	300	5	1	NA	25	830	55
Scrambled Eggs	3 oz.	160	12	3	NA	405	100	NA
Biscuit	1 item	370	23	5	NA	0	890	35
Croissant	1 item	210	10	4	NA	5	200	26
Cinnamon 'n Raisin Biscuit	1 item	280	12	3	NA	0	650	NA
Grits	5 oz.	110	5	1	NA	0	480	NA
Hash Rounds (small)	3 oz.	260	16	4	NA	0	360	25
Breakfast Items								
Bacon Biscuit	1 item	430	28	7	NA	10	1110	35
Bacon, Egg & Cheese Biscuit	1 item	560	38	11	NA	225	1360	37
Sausage Biscuit	1 item	530	38	10	NA	30	1240	36
Sausage & Egg Biscuit	1 item	610	44	11	NA	235	1290	36
Country Ham Biscuit	1 item	430	28	7	NA	10	1110	36
Bacon, Egg & Cheese Biscuit	1 item	560	38	11	NA	225	1360	37
Ham, Egg & Cheese Biscuit	1 item	560	35	10	NA	245	1800	37
Smoked Sausage Biscuit	1 item	620	46	15	NA	40	1680	NA
Chicken Fillet Biscuit	1 item	600	34	7	NA	55	1680	50
Country Steak Biscuit	1 item	620	41	11	NA	35	1360	44
Loaded Omelette Biscuit	1 item	640	44	14	NA	245	1510	37
Sunrise Croissant w/ bacon	1 item	450	29	12	NA	240	900	28
Sunrise Croissant w/ ham	1 item	430	26	10	NA	250	1050	28
Sunrise Croissant w/ sausage	1 item	550	38	15	NA	265	1030	29
Frisco Breakfast item	1 item	410	17	7	NA	245	870	37
Tortilla Scrambler	1 item	230	13	6	NA	30	520	NA

Hardee's®
Continued

Thickburgers

	Serving	Calories	Total fat (gm)	Saturated fat (gm)	Trans fats (gm)	Cholesterol (mg)	Sodium (mg)	Carbs (gm)
Thickburger	1 item	850	57	22	NA	105	1470	53
Cheeseburger	1 item	680	39	19	NA	90	1450	52
Bacon Cheese Thickburger	1 item	910	63	24	NA	115	1490	50
Chili Cheese Thickburger	1 item	870	54	26	NA	135	1840	NA
Mushroom 'n Swiss Thickburger	1 item	720	42	21	NA	100	1570	48
Monster Thickburger	1 item	1420	108	43	NA	230	2770	46
Low-Carb Thickburger	1 item	420	32	12	NA	115	1010	5
Six Dollar Burger	1 item	1060	72	30	NA	150	1860	58
Grilled Sourdough	1 item	1040	73	30	NA	155	1420	42

Other Items

	Serving	Calories	Total fat (gm)	Saturated fat (gm)	Trans fats (gm)	Cholesterol (mg)	Sodium (mg)	Carbs (gm)
Slammer	1 item	240	12	5	NA	35	300	NA
Slammer w/ cheese	1 item	280	16	8	NA	45	500	NA
Big Chicken item	1 item	770	36	8	NA	95	2000	76
Charbroiled Chicken Sandwich	1 item	590	26	7	NA	80	1180	32
Charbroiled BBQ Chicken Sandwich	1 item	340	4	1	NA	60	1070	40
Low-Carb Charbroiled Chicken Club	1 item	420	24	7	NA	95	1230	10
Spicy Chicken Sandwich	1 item	470	26	5	NA	40	1220	46
Regular Roast Beef	1 item	330	16	7	NA	40	860	29
Big Roast Beef	1 item	470	23	10	NA	60	1290	38
Hot Ham 'n Cheese	1 item	287	13	6	NA	37	1110	39
Big Hot Ham 'n Cheese	1 item	485	20	10	NA	74	2009	40
Hot Dog	1 item	420	30	12	NA	55	1200	22
Chicken Strips	3 items	380	21	4	NA	55	1360	27

Kid's Meals

	Serving	Calories	Total fat (gm)	Saturated fat (gm)	Trans fats (gm)	Cholesterol (mg)	Sodium (mg)	Carbs (gm)
Slammer	1 meal	720	35	13	NA	70	740	NA
Chicken Strips w/o sauce	1 meal	500	25	5	NA	35	1050	50
French Fries	3 oz.	250	12	3	NA	0	150	32

Fried Chicken

	Serving	Calories	Total fat (gm)	Saturated fat (gm)	Trans fats (gm)	Cholesterol (mg)	Sodium (mg)	Carbs (gm)
Breast	1 item	370	15	4	NA	75	1190	29
Wing	1 item	200	8	2	NA	30	740	23
Thigh	1 item	330	15	4	NA	60	1000	30
Leg	1 item	170	7	2	NA	45	570	15

Side Items

	Serving	Calories	Total fat (gm)	Saturated fat (gm)	Trans fats (gm)	Cholesterol (mg)	Sodium (mg)	Carbs (gm)
French Fries (small)	4.5 oz.	390	19	4	NA	0	240	51
Crispy Curls	4 oz.	340	17	4	NA	0	840	43
Chili Cheese Fries	9 oz.	700	39	13	NA	50	780	NA
Cole Slaw	4 oz.	170	10	2	NA	10	140	20

Hardee's®
Continued
Side Items continued

	Serving	Calories	Total fat (gm)	Saturated fat (gm)	Trans fats (gm)	Cholesterol (mg)	Sodium (mg)	Carbs (gm)
Mashed Potatoes (small)	5 oz.	90	2	0	NA	0	410	17
Chicken Gravy	1.5 oz.	20	1	0	NA	0	220	3

Hometown Buffet®
Breads & Other Items

	Serving	Calories	Total fat (gm)	Saturated fat (gm)	Trans fats (gm)	Cholesterol (mg)	Sodium (mg)	Carbs (gm)
Biscuits	1 item	180	7	2	NA	0	450	24
Breadsticks	1 item	140	5	1	NA	0	260	21
Buns, Hot Dog	1 bun	120	2	1	NA	0	240	22
Cinnamon Bread	1 slice	45	1	0	NA	0	30	10
Cinnamon Sugared Donut Holes	1 item	50	3	1	NA	0	75	5
Dinner Roll, Wheat	1 roll	110	3	1	NA	0	160	18
Dinner Roll, White	1 roll	120	4	1	NA	0	200	20
English Muffin	½	60	1	0	NA	0	130	13
Flour Tortilla	1 item	120	3	1	NA	0	240	20
French Toast	1 slice	170	8	2	NA	100	190	24
Glazed Donuts	1 item	130	7	2	NA	0	40	16
Pancakes	1 item	120	4	1	NA	0	280	19
Taco Shells	1 shell	50	3	1	NA	0	0	7
Waffles	1 item	120	3	1	NA	0	440	19

Dessert Items

	Serving	Calories	Total fat (gm)	Saturated fat (gm)	Trans fats (gm)	Cholesterol (mg)	Sodium (mg)	Carbs (gm)
Apple Crisp	1 spoon	150	4	1	NA	0	95	31
Bread Pudding	1 spoon	190	8	4	NA	35	130	27
Butterfinger Pieces	1 spoon	70	3	2	NA	0	35	11
Cheesecake (plain)	1 item	220	10	5	NA	0	180	29
Chocolate Chips	1 spoon	90	5	4	NA	0	0	10
Chocolate Cream Pie Reduced-Sugar	1 item	190	12	8	NA	0	140	18
Chocolate Decadence Cake	1 item	200	9	4	NA	30	200	27
Cone, Ice Cream	1 cone	15	0	0	NA	0	15	3
Pudding, Chocolate	1 spoon	150	7	1	NA	0	130	19
Pudding, Chocolate Reduced-Sugar/Calorie	1 spoon	70	1	1	NA	0	270	14
Pudding, Vanilla	1 spoon	140	6	6	NA	0	115	19
Pudding, Vanilla Reduced-Sugar/Calorie	1 spoon	70	1	1	NA	0	260	14
Pumpkin pie	1 item	270	6	3	NA	50	230	31
Reduced-Sugar Pie–Apple	1 item	190	11	2	NA	0	250	24

Hometown Buffet® Continued

Dessert Items continued

	Serving	Calories	Total fat (gm)	Saturated fat (gm)	Trans fats (gm)	Cholesterol (mg)	Sodium (mg)	Carbs (gm)
Reduced-Sugar Pie–Cherry	1 item	160	9	6	NA	0	230	16
Reduced-Sugar Pie–Lemon	1 item	160	9	6	NA	0	230	16
Reduced-Sugar Pie–Lime	1 item	160	9	6	NA	0	230	16
Reduced-Sugar Pie–Orange	1 item	160	9	6	NA	0	230	16
Reduced-Sugar Pie–Raspberry	1 item	160	9	6	NA	0	230	16
Reduced-Sugar Pie–Strawberry	1 item	160	9	6	NA	0	230	16
Soft Serve Frozen Yogurt, Non-fat, Strawberry	4 fl. oz.	100	0	0	NA	0	70	23
Soft Serve Frozen Yogurt, Non-Fat, Vanilla	4 fl. oz.	110	0	0	NA	0	75	23
Soft Serve, Chocolate	4 fl. oz.	140	5	3	NA	20	120	24
Soft Serve, Vanilla	4 fl. oz.	150	5	3	NA	25	115	25
Semi Sweet Frozen Yogurt, Non-Fat, Nutrasweet, Vanilla	4 fl. oz.	80	0	0	NA	0	80	17

Entrées

	Serving	Calories	Total fat (gm)	Saturated fat (gm)	Trans fats (gm)	Cholesterol (mg)	Sodium (mg)	Carbs (gm)
BBQ Beef Ribs	1 order	300	23	9	NA	60	350	7
BBQ Smoked Sausage	1 spoon	140	10	4	NA	10	380	9
Beef Liver & Onion	1 item	80	3	1	NA	160	190	4
Carved Beef Brisket	3 oz.	200	11	4	NA	80	470	1
Carved Ham	3 oz.	140	9	3	NA	45	970	0
Carved Peppered Pork Loin	3 oz.	160	8	4	NA	60	810	0
Carved Roast Beef	3 oz.	230	15	7	NA	70	55	0
Carved Roast Turkey	3 oz.	170	8	3	NA	70	60	0
Carved Salmon Fillet	3 oz.	190	12	2	NA	60	390	0
Chicken & Dumplings	1 spoon	190	7	2	NA	20	710	24
Chicken Cacciatore	1 spoon	220	11	3	NA	95	320	3
Chicken, Hand Breaded Fried–breast	1 breast	310	16	5	NA	150	470	3
Chicken, Hand Breaded Fried–drumstick	1 drumstick	90	6	2	NA	50	110	2
Chicken, Hand Breaded Fried–thigh	1 thigh	210	14	4	NA	115	250	4
Chicken, Traditional Baked–breast	1 breast	280	12	4	NA	125	230	0
Chicken, Traditional Baked–drumstick	1 drumstick	90	6	2	NA	35	100	0
Chicken, Traditional Baked–thigh	1 thigh	160	11	3	NA	60	180	0
Chinese Chicken Livers	1 spoon	200	12	2	NA	135	340	17
Country BBQ Chicken–breast	1 breast	300	12	4	NA	125	370	5
Country BBQ Chicken–drumstick	1 drumstick	110	6	2	NA	35	190	3
Country BBQ Chicken–thigh	1 thigh	210	13	4	NA	75	245	4
Country BBQ Chicken–wing	1 wing	70	3	1	NA	25	180	3
Denver Scrambled Eggs	1 spoon	140	11	3	NA	240	220	2

Entrées continued

	Serving	Calories	Total fat (gm)	Saturated fat (gm)	Trans fats (gm)	Cholesterol (mg)	Sodium (mg)	Carbs (gm)
Egg, Poached	1 item	70	5	2	NA	210	150	0
Eggs Benedict	1 item	250	15	4	NA	225	840	15
Fish Patties	1 item	160	9	2	NA	25	430	13
Fish, Fried	1 item	80	4	1	NA	10	130	9
Hamburger Patties	1 item	220	19	13	NA	40	140	0
Hot Dogs, Turkey	1 hot dog	130	11	4	NA	50	570	2
Hot Wings–Drummies	1 drummie	35	2	1	NA	20	140	0
Hot Wings–Wing	1 wing	25	2	1	NA	15	110	0
Mini Corn Dog	1 item	50	2	1	NA	10	60	6
Mostaciolli	1 spoon	120	5	2	NA	10	320	13
Orange Chicken	1 spoon	240	11	3	NA	45	510	24
Quiche, Breakfast	1 spoon	220	15	5	NA	120	450	12
Scrambled Eggs	1 spoon	130	11	3	NA	250	80	0
Shrimp, Fried	6 shrimp	110	5	1	NA	35	270	11
Sauerkraut	1 spoon	5	0	0	NA	0	110	1
Smoked Sausage & Sauerkraut (sausage only)	1 link	190	17	8	NA	25	460	2
Spanish Rice	1 spoon	140	9	4	NA	20	280	9
Taco Meat, Beef	2 fl. oz.	100	5	2	NA	30	310	3
Teriyaki Chicken Wings-Drummies	1 drummie	50	3	1	NA	20	135	2
Teriyaki Chicken Wings-Wing	1 wing	50	3	1	NA	10	130	2

Fruits (seasonal)

	Serving	Calories	Total fat (gm)	Saturated fat (gm)	Trans fats (gm)	Cholesterol (mg)	Sodium (mg)	Carbs (gm)
Cantaloupe	1 spoon	25	0	0	NA	0	10	6
Grapes	1 spoon	60	0	0	NA	0	0	15
Honeydew	1 spoon	30	0	0	NA	0	15	8
Pineapple	1 spoon	35	0	0	NA	0	0	10
Strawberries	1 spoon	25	0	0	NA	0	0	6
Watermelon	1 spoon	25	0	0	NA	0	0	6

Side Items

	Serving	Calories	Total fat (gm)	Saturated fat (gm)	Trans fats (gm)	Cholesterol (mg)	Sodium (mg)	Carbs (gm)
Bacon	1 slice	30	3	1	NA	10	145	0
Baked Beans	1 spoon	120	1	0	NA	0	530	29
Bread Dressing	1 spoon	130	4	1	NA	10	460	21
Cabbage, German Boiled	1 spoon	40	4	1	NA	0	150	3
Cabbage, Green	1 spoon	40	3	1	NA	0	110	3
Carrots, Steamed	1 spoon	40	0	0	NA	0	45	9
Chesapeake Corn	1 spoon	80	3	1	NA	0	210	13
Corn on the Cob	1 item	100	3	1	NA	0	0	16
Corn, Steamed	1 spoon	100	1	0	NA	0	210	21
Creamy Cheese Sauce	2 fl oz	50	2	1	NA	2	630	9

Hometown Buffet
Continued
Side Items continued

	Serving	Calories	Total fat (gm)	Saturated fat (gm)	Trans fats (gm)	Cholesterol (mg)	Sodium (mg)	Carbs (gm)
French Fries	22 fries	190	9	2	NA	0	380	24
Fried Rice w/ ham	1 spoon	170	6	2	NA	75	640	23
Green Bean Casserole	1 spoon	60	3	1	NA	0	210	9
Green Beans	1 spoon	15	0	0	NA	0	250	3
Green Beans El Greco	1 spoon	20	0	0	NA	0	170	5
Grits	4 fl oz	70	0	0	NA	0	270	16
Italian Style Green Beans w/ bacon	1 spoon	60	4	1	NA	0	280	NA
Joe's Cracked Pepper Green Beans	1 spoon	70	6	2	NA	10	240	5
Montreal Vegetable Medley	1 spoon	40	4	1	NA	0	110	3
Oatmeal	4 fl. oz.	70	1	0	NA	0	120	13
Pinto Beans w/ ham	1 spoon	90	1	0	NA	0	370	21
Potatoes, Baked	1 items	160	0	0	NA	0	10	39
Potatoes, Baked Sweet	1 items	160	0	0	NA	0	54	47
Potatoes, Hash Browns	1 spoon	110	6	1	NA	0	140	13
Potatoes, Hash Brown Patties	1 item	120	8	3	NA	0	200	11
Potatoes, Jo Jo	6-7 items	210	15	4	NA	5	210	18
Potatoes, O'Brien	1 spoon	120	6	1	NA	0	210	16
Potatoes, Red	1 spoon	100	3	1	NA	0	10	18
Red Beans w/ ham	1 spoon	60	1	0	NA	0	440	18
Sausage Links	1 link	100	10	4	NA	30	170	0
Spaghetti	1 spoon	60	1	0	NA	0	90	19
Spinach Marie	1 spoon	210	17	6	NA	140	420	8
Squash, Winter	1 spoon	150	9	2	NA	0	10	18
Turnip or Collard Greens w/ bacon	1 spoon	40	3	1	NA	0	310	2
Vegetable Stir Fry	1 spoon	25	1	0	NA	0	180	6
White Rice	1 spoon	90	0	0	NA	0	300	22
Wild Rice Vegetable Pilaf	1 spoon	90	1	0	NA	0	370	17
Yams, Candied	1 spoon	140	2	0	NA	0	55	30
Zucchini, Sautéed	1 spoon	50	4	1	NA	0	55	3
Soups								
Chicken Noodle Soup	4 fl. oz.	70	2	1	NA	30	360	7
Chicken Rice Soup	4 fl. oz.	70	2	1	NA	25	360	8
Chili Bean Soup	4 fl. oz.	100	4	1	NA	20	370	9
Corn Chowder	4 fl. oz.	140	8	5	NA	0	310	15
Cream of Broccoli Soup	4 fl. oz.	80	7	4	NA	0	250	5
Navy Bean Soup w/ ham	4 fl. oz.	50	1	0	NA	0	410	10
New England Clam Chowder	4 fl. oz.	300	12	8	NA	5	580	9
Potato Cheese Soup	4 fl. oz.	130	9	5	NA	10	270	11

I Can't Believe It's Yogurt!®

	Serving	Calories	Total fat (gm)	Saturated fat (gm)	Trans fats (gm)	Cholesterol (mg)	Sodium (mg)	Carbs (gm)
Original Frozen Yogurt								
Awesome Amaretto	½ cup	130	3	2	0	10	105	NA
Cookies 'n Cream	½ cup	120	2	1	0	5	90	NA
Peanut Butter Bliss	½ cup	140	6	2	0	5	95	NA
French Vanilla	½ cup	120	3	2	0	20	90	NA
Non-fat Frozen Yogurt								
Various Flavors	½ cup	100	0	0	0	0	70	NA
Non-fat w/ NutraSweet® Frozen Yogurt								
Chocolicious	½ cup	100	0	0	0	0	70	NA
Various Flavors	½ cup	90	0	0	0	0	75	NA
Hand-Scooped Frozen Yogurt								
Amaretto Cherry Crunch	½ cup	170	5	2	0	25	95	NA
Chunky Chocolate Brownie	½ cup	180	6	3	0	10	135	NA
Chocolate Chip Cookie Dough	½ cup	180	5	3	0	40	120	NA
Cookies & Cream	½ cup	170	5	3	0	25	120	NA
Rocky Road	½ cup	180	6	3	0	10	125	NA
Classic Vanilla	½ cup	160	4	2	0	40	115	NA
Yoglace Frozen Dairy Dessert								
Various Flavors	½ cup	45	0	0	0	5	30	NA

IHOP® (International House of Pancakes®)
Does not provide nutrition information.

Hooters®
Does not provide nutrition information.

NOTES:

_____

_____

_____

_____

In-N-Out Burger®

	Serving	Calories	Total fat (gm)	Saturated fat (gm)	Trans fats (gm)	Cholesterol (mg)	Sodium (mg)	Carbs (gm)
Hamburgers								
Hamburger w/ onion	1 item	390	19	5	0	40	650	39
Hamburger w/ mustard & ketchup instead of spread	1 item	310	10	4	0	35	730	41
Protein-Style Hamburger	1 item	240	17	4	0	40	370	11
Cheeseburger w/ onion	1 item	480	27	10	0.5	60	1000	39
Cheeseburger w/ mustard & ketchup instead of spread	1 item	400	18	9	0.5	60	1080	41
Protein-Style Cheeseburger	1 item	330	25	9	0.5	60	720	11
Double-Double w/ onion	1 item	670	41	18	1	120	1440	39
Double-Double w/ mustard & ketchup instead of spread	1 item	590	32	17	1	115	1520	41
Protein-Style Double-Double	1 item	520	39	17	1	120	1160	11
French Fries								
French Fries	4.5 oz.	400	18	5	0	0	245	54
Shakes								
Chocolate	15 fl. oz.	690	36	24	0	95	350	83
Strawberry	15 fl. oz.	690	33	22	0	85	280	91
Vanilla	15 fl. oz.	680	37	25	0	90	390	78

Jack in the Box®

	Serving	Calories	Total fat (gm)	Saturated fat (gm)	Trans fats (gm)	Cholesterol (mg)	Sodium (mg)	Carbs (gm)
Breakfast								
Bacon Breakfast Jack	1 item	300	14	5	1	215	730	29
Bacon, Egg, & Cheese Biscuit	1 item	430	25	8	5	220	110	34
Blueberry French Toast Sticks	1 item	450	20	5	5	0	550	59
Breakfast Jack	1 item	305	14	4	2	205	715	29
Chicken Biscuit	1 item	450	24	6	6	30	980	42
Ciabatta Breakfast Sandwich	1 item	710	36	10	1	440	1730	63
Extreme Sausage item	1 item	690	50	17	1.5	280	1265	31
Meaty Breakfast Burrito	1 item	480	29	10	1	350	1210	29
Original French Toast Sticks	1 item	470	23	5	5	25	450	58
Sourdough Breakfast item	1 item	445	26	8	2	215	875	NA
Ultimate Breakfast item	1 item	605	31	10	2	425	1630	49
Sausage Breakfast Jack	1 item	450	28	10	1	245	840	29
Sausage Biscuit	1 item	600	36	9	7	35	1200	32
Sausage, Egg & Cheese Biscuit	1 item	970	68	21	8	280	1905	35
Sausage Croissant	1 item	605	41	13	4	240	725	37
Sirloin Steak and Egg Burrito	1 item	790	48	15	4	450	1320	52
Spicy Chicken Biscuit	1 item	460	22	5	7	40	1020	44
Supreme Croissant	1 item	475	27	9	4	220	815	36
Hash Browns	2 oz.	150	10	3	3	0	230	13

Jack in the Box®
Continued

	Serving	Calories	Total fat (gm)	Saturated fat (gm)	Trans fats (gm)	Cholesterol (mg)	Sodium (mg)	Carbs (gm)
Burgers								
Hamburger	1 item	310	14	5	0	45	590	30
Hamburger w/ cheese	1 item	355	18	7	0	55	770	31
Hamburger Deluxe	1 item	370	21	6	0	50	545	31
Hamburger Deluxe w/ cheese	1 item	460	28	10	0	75	915	33
Jumbo Jack	1 item	600	35	12	1	45	935	51
Jumbo Jack w/ cheese	1 item	695	42	16	1	70	1305	54
Junior Bacon Cheeseburger	1 item	525	36	10	0	70	880	30
Sourdough Jack	1 item	715	51	18	3	75	1165	36
Bacon Bacon Cheeseburger	1 item	780	50	19	1	90	1545	NA
Bacon 'n Cheese Ciabatta Burger	1 item	1120	76	28	3	135	167	66
Sirloin Cheese Burger	1 item	1070	71	25	2	180	1850	61
Sirloin Bacon & Cheese Burger	1 item	1120	76	24	3	190	2620	63
Ultimate Cheeseburger	1 item	945	65	27	3	120	1525	53
Bacon Ultimate Cheeseburger	1 item	1025	71	29	3	135	1985	53
Chicken & Fish								
Jack's Spicy Chicken	1 item	615	31	6	3	50	1090	61
Jack's Spicy Chicken w/ cheese	1 item	695	37	10	3	70	1400	62
Chicken item	1 item	390	21	4	2	35	730	38
Chicken item w/ cheese	1 item	430	24	6	2	45	880	NA
Chipotle Chicken Ciabatta w/ Grilled Chicen	1 item	690	28	9	0	105	1850	65
Chipotle Chicken Ciabatta w/ Spciy Crispy Chicken	1 item	750	34	10	3	80	1650	75
Bacon Chicken item	1 item	440	24	6	3	40	970	39
Chicken Cordon Bleu	1 item	555	28	9	2	100	1335	NA
Sirloin Steak & Cheddar Ciabatta	1 item	770	38	8	0	110	1310	65
Sourdough Grilled Chicken Club	1 item	505	27	7	2	75	1220	34
Classic Chicken Ciabatta	1 item	510	13	3	0	65	1700	NA
Bruschetta Chicken Ciabatta	1 item	660	26	7	0	85	1880	67
Chicken Fajita Pita	1 item	315	9	4	0	65	1080	30
Southwest Pita	1 item	260	5	1	0	40	880	NA
Chicken Breast Strips	8 oz.	630	38	8	6	90	1470	36
Fish & Chips (large)	1 meal	840	56	11	10	55	1600	92
Tacos & Snacks								
Bacon Cheddar Potato Wedges	1 item	720	48	15	12	45	1360	52
Fruit Cup	1 item	90	0	0	0	0	20	22
Egg Roll	1 item	175	6	2	1	5	470	15
Mozarella Cheese Sticks	3 items	240	12	5	2	25	420	21
Sampler Trio	1 item	750	39	14	7	85	1760	65
Spicy Chicken Bites	7 pieces	290	14	3	3	45	660	21

Jack in the Box®
Continued

Tacos & Snacks continued	Serving	Calories	Total fat (gm)	Saturated fat (gm)	Trans fats (gm)	Cholesterol (mg)	Sodium (mg)	Carbs (gm)
Stuffed Jalapeños	3 items	230	13	6	2	20	690	22
Taco	1 taco	160	8	3	1	15	270	15
Monster Taco	1 taco	240	14	5	2	20	390	20
Items								
Ultimate Club item	1 item	630	29	9	0	105	1985	NA
Deli Trio Pannido	1 item	645	34	9	0	95	2530	NA
Ham & Turkey Pannido	1 item	610	29	7	0	110	1785	NA
Zesty Turkey Pannido	1 item	740	44	11	0	135	1880	NA
Salads (w/ dressing unless noted)								
Asian Grilled Chicken Salad	1 salad	160	1.5	0	0	65	380	18
Asian Crispy Chicken Salad	1 salad	330	13	3	3	40	650	34
Grilled Chicken Club Salad	1 salad	320	16	6	0	105	780	28
Crispy Chicken Club Salad	1 salad	480	27	9	3	80	1060	5
Southwest Grilled Chicken Salad	1 salad	320	12	6	0	90	760	27
Southwest Crispy Chicken Salad	1 salad	480	23	8	3	70	1040	44
Side Salad w/o dressing	1 salad	155	8	3	2	10	290	5
Side Items								
French Fries (small)	3.5 oz.	270	12	3	4	0	440	41
Seasoned Curly Fries (small)	3 oz.	270	15	3	5	0	590	30
Onion Rings	4.5 oz.	500	30	6	10	0	420	51

Joe's Crab Shack®
Does not provide nutrition information.

KFC®

Original Recipe Chicken	Serving	Calories	Total fat (gm)	Saturated fat (gm)	Trans fats (gm)	Cholesterol (mg)	Sodium (mg)	Carbs (gm)
Breast	1 item	360	21	5	0	115	1020	7
Breast w/o skin	1 item	140	2	0	0	65	520	1
Drumstick	1 item	130	8	2	0	65	350	2
Thigh	1 item	330	24	6	0	110	870	8
Whole Wing	1 item	130	8	2	0	50	350	4
Extra Crispy Chicken								
Breast	1 item	440	27	6	0	105	970	15
Drumstick	1 item	160	10	2	0	55	370	6
Thigh	1 item	370	28	6	0	85	850	12
Whole Wing	1 item	170	11	2.5	0	55	350	6

	Serving	Calories	Total fat (gm)	Saturated fat (gm)	Trans fats (gm)	Cholesterol (mg)	Sodium (mg)	Carbs (gm)
Other Chicken Specialties								
Chicken Pot Pie	1 item	770	40	15	14	115	1680	70
Crispy Strips	2 items	240	13	2.5	0	50	800	11
Crispy Strips	3 items	350	19	3.5	0	70	1190	16
Popcorn Chicken (kids)	1 item	290	19	3.5	0	40	850	16
Popcorn Chicken (individual)	1 item	400	26	4.5	0	60	1160	22
Popcorn Chicken (large)	1 item	550	35	6	0	80	1600	30
Honey BBQ Wings	5 items	390	24	5	0	105	830	23
Boneless Honey BBQ Wings	5 items	450	20	3.5	0	65	1880	41
Fiery Buffalo Wings	5 items	380	24	5	0	105	1480	19
Boneless Firey Buffalo Wings	5 items	420	20	3.5	0	65	2260	33
Sweet & Spicy Wings	5 items	400	24	5	0	105	760	24
Boneless Sweet & Spicy Wings	5 items	440	19	3.5	0	65	1700	38
Teriyaki Wings	5 Pieces	480	25	5	0	105	830	40
Boneless Teriyaki Wings	5 Pieces	500	21	4	0	65	1730	50
Hot Wings	5 items	350	24	5	0	105	740	14
Salads (w/o dressing or croutons)								
Roasted Caesar	1 salad	220	8	4.5	0	70	830	6
Crispy Caesar	1 salad	350	19	6	0	70	1080	16
Caesar Side	1 salad	50	3	2	0	10	135	2
Roasted BLT	1 salad	200	6	2	0	65	880	8
Crispy BLT	1 salad	330	17	4	0	65	1130	18
House Side	1 salad	15	0	0	0	0	10	2
Side Choices								
Baked Beans	5 oz.	220	1	0	0	0	730	45
Baked Cheetos	1 item	120	4.5	1	0	0	210	NA
Biscuit w/ butter	1 item	220	11	2.5	3.5	0	640	24
Corn on the Cob (small)	1 item	70	1.5	0.5	0	0	5	13
Corn on the Cob (large)	1 item	150	3	1	0	0	10	26
Cole Slaw	4.5 oz.	180	10	1.5	0	5	270	22
Green Beans	3.5 oz.	50	1.5	0	0	5	570	7
Macaroni & Cheese	5 oz.	180	8	3.5	1	15	800	18
Potato Salad	4.5 oz	180	9	1.5	0	5	470	22
Famous Bowl Rice w/ gravy	14 oz.	620	28	7	1	60	2150	67
Famous Bowl Mashed Potatoes w/ gravy	19 oz.	740	35	9	1.5	60	2350	80
Mashed Potatoes w/o gravy	4 oz.	110	4	1	0	0	320	17
Mashed Potatoes w/ gravy	5 oz.	140	5	1	0.5	0	560	20
Potato Wedges (small)	3.5 oz.	260	13	2.5	0	0	740	33
Sandwiches								
KFC Snacker	1 item	320	16	3	0	30	680	29
KFC Snacker, Buffalo	1 item	260	8	1.5	0	25	860	31

KFC® Continued	Serving	Calories	Total fat (gm)	Saturated fat (gm)	Trans fats (gm)	Cholesterol (mg)	Sodium (mg)	Carbs (gm)
KFC Snacker, Fish	1 item	330	15	3	0	60	710	31
KFC Snacker, Ultimate Cheese	1 item	280	11	2.5	0.5	25	780	30
Sandwiches continued								
KFC Snacker, Honey BBQ	1 item	210	3	0.5	0	40	530	32
Honey BBQ	1 item	280	3.5	0	0	60	780	32
Double Crunch	1 item	470	23	5	0	55	1190	38
Crispy Twister	1 item	600	33	0	0	55	1500	49
Oven Roasted Twister	1 item	470	23	0	0	60	1260	40
Oven Roasted Twister w/o sauce	1 item	330	7	0	0	50	1120	39
Tender Roast	1 item	430	18	0	0	80	1180	29
Tender Roast w/o sauce	1 item	300	4.5	0	0	70	1060	28
Desserts								
Quaker Chewy S'mores Granola Bar	1 item	100	2	0.5	0	0	80	NA
Apple Pie Mini's	3 items	370	20	6	0	0	260	44
Double Chocolate Chip Cake	1 item	330	16	4	1	50	200	41
Lil' Bucket Fudge Brownie	1 item	280	11	4	0.5	20	200	NA
Lil' Bucket Lemon Créme	1 item	410	15	7	1.5	0	270	61
Lil' Bucket Chocolate Créme	1 item	280	13	9	1	0	230	38
Lil' Bucket Strawberry Shortcake	1 item	210	7	5	0	10	125	33
Sweet Life Sugar Cookie	1 item	160	6	2.5	0	5	120	23
Sweet Life Oatmeal Raisin Cookie	1 item	150	5	2.5	0	5	135	24
Sweet Life Chocolate Chip Cookie	1 item	160	7	3.5	0	10	95	23

Fast Food Factoid:

Taste, cost, and convenience are the main reasons many people struggle to eat good fast foods. Try a GREEN food—you might be surprised.

NOTES:

_____

_____

_____

_____

Krispy Kreme®

Doughnuts	Serving	Calories	Total fat (gm)	Saturated fat (gm)	Trans fats (gm)	Cholesterol (mg)	Sodium (mg)	Carbs (gm)
Original Glazed	52 g	200	12	3	4	5	95	22
Chocolate Iced Glazed	66 g	250	12	3	4	5	100	33
Chocolate Iced w/ sprinkles	71 g	260	12	3	4	5	100	38
Chocolate Iced Kreme Filled	86 g	350	20	5	6	5	140	38
Chocolate Iced Custard Filled	86 g	300	17	4	5	5	140	35
Glazed Lemon Filled	85 g	290	16	4	5	5	135	35
Glazed Raspberry Filled	85 g	300	16	4	5	5	125	38
Glazed Cruller	54 g	240	14	4	4.5	15	240	26
Cinnamon Apple Filled	81 g	290	16	4	5	5	150	32
New York Cheesecake	90 g	320	19	5	6	10	190	35
Caramel Kreme Crunch	92 g	350	19	5	6	5	170	46
Key Lime Pie	92 g	320	17	5	5	5	1050	40
Glazed Chocolate Cake	81 g	300	15	4	5	5	310	41
Traditional Cake	57 g	230	13	3	4	20	320	25
Glazed Kreme Filled	86 g	340	20	5	6	5	140	38
Glazed Blueberry	80 g	330	17	4	5	20	290	43
Glazed Cinnamon	54 g	210	12	3	4	5	100	24
Cinnamon Bun	67 g	260	16	4	5	5	125	28
Cinnamon Twist	59 g	230	9	3	5	5	85	23
Maple Iced Glaze	66 g	240	12	3	5	5	100	32
Glazed Sour Cream	80 g	340	18	5	4	20	310	42
Sugar	49 g	200	12	3	4	5	95	21
Powdered Blueberry Filled	81 g	290	16	4	NA	5	140	NA
Powdered Strawberry Filled	81 g	290	16	4	5	5	135	33
Powdered Cake	71 g	280	14	3	4	20	320	37
Chocolate Iced Cake	71 g	270	14	3	4	20	320	36
Chocolate Glazed Cruller	69 g	290	15	4	4.5	15	240	37
Dulce De Leche	75 g	290	18	5	5	5	160	30
Apple Fritter	108 g	400	24	6	7	10	135	46
Whole Wheat Glazed	48 g	180	11	3	3.5	5	100	19
Doughnut Holes								
Original Glazed Doughnut Holes	5 items	200	17	3	NA	5	95	25
Glazed Blueberry Doughnut Holes	4 items	220	19	3	NA	20	270	26
Glazed Cake Doughnut Holes	4 items	210	16	3	NA	15	230	28
Glazed Chocolate Cake Doughnut Holes	4 items	210	16	3	NA	15	230	28
Frozen Blends (does not include whipped cream topping)								
Frozen Raspberry Blend	12 oz.	430	13	10	NA	25	160	NA
Frozen Raspberry Blend	16 oz.	590	19	15	NA	35	230	NA
Frozen Raspberry Blend	20 oz.	710	22	17	NA	35	270	NA
Frozen Original Kreme Blend	12 oz.	440	15	12	NA	25	200	NA

Krispy Kreme®
Continued

Frozen Blends (does not include whipped cream topping) continued

	Serving	Calories	Total fat (gm)	Saturated fat (gm)	Trans fats (gm)	Cholesterol (mg)	Sodium (mg)	Carbs (gm)
Frozen Original Kreme Blend	16 oz.	600	21	17	NA	35	270	NA
Frozen Original Kreme Blend	20 oz.	730	24	20	NA	35	330	NA
Frozen Original Kreme w/ coffee blend	12 oz.	440	15	12	NA	25	210	NA
Frozen Original Kreme w/ coffee blend	16 oz.	600	21	17	NA	35	280	NA
Frozen Original Kreme w/ coffee blend	20 oz.	730	24	20	NA	35	340	NA
Frozen Latte Blend	12 oz.	440	16	13	NA	25	210	NA
Frozen Latte Blend	16 oz.	610	22	18	NA	35	280	NA
Frozen Latte Blend	20 oz.	740	26	21	NA	35	340	NA
Frozen Double Chocolate Blend	12 oz.	440	16	11	NA	25	210	NA
Frozen Double Chocolate Blend	16 oz.	610	22	16	NA	35	280	NA
Frozen Double Chocolate Blend	20 oz.	740	26	18	NA	35	340	NA
Frozen Double Chocolate w/ coffee blend	12 oz.	440	16	10	NA	25	210	NA
Frozen Double Chocolate w/ coffee blend	16 oz.	600	22	15	NA	35	280	NA
Frozen Double Chocolate w/ coffee blend	20 oz.	730	26	17	NA	35	340	NA
Reduced-Calorie Double Chocolate Blend	12 oz.	99	1	0	NA	2	104	NA
Reduced-Calorie Latte Blend	12 oz.	99	1	0	NA	2	117	NA

Fast Food Factoid:
Chronic diseases don't just happen; they are almost entirely the result of decades of unhealthy living.
Dr. Steven Aldana, The Culprit and The Cure

Krystal®
Breakfast

	Serving	Calories	Total fat (gm)	Saturated fat (gm)	Trans fats (gm)	Cholesterol (mg)	Sodium (mg)	Carbs (gm)
Sunriser	1 item	240	14	5	NA	255	460	14
Biscuit & Gravy	7 oz.	280	14	3	NA	0	710	34
Sausage Biscuit	1 item	480	33	10	NA	40	980	33
Bacon, Egg & Cheese Biscuit	1 item	390	23	7	NA	40	1090	33
Chik Biscuit	1 item	360	15	3	NA	20	1030	40
Kryspers	2 oz.	190	13	5	NA	10	340	17
Country Breakfast	1 meal	660	42	14	NA	590	1450	46
Plain Biscuit	1 biscuit	270	13	3	0	0	660	33
Scrambler	1 meal	440	26	11	NA	255	840	33
4 Carb Scrambler w/ bacon	5.5 oz.	370	29	10	1	595	830	4
4 Carb Scrambler w/ sausage	7.5 oz.	600	51	18	2	600	1040	3

Krystal® Continued

Hamburgers

	Serving	Calories	Total fat (gm)	Saturated fat (gm)	Trans fats (gm)	Cholesterol (mg)	Sodium (mg)	Carbs (gm)
Krystal	1 item	160	7	3	NA	20	260	17
Double Krystal	1 item	260	13	6	NA	40	550	24
Cheese Krystal	1 item	180	9	4	NA	25	430	17
Double Cheese Krystal	1 item	310	16	7	NA	65	800	26
Bacon Cheese Krystal	1 item	190	10	5	NA	25	430	16
B.A. Burger	1 item	470	27	8	1	55	760	39
B.A. Burger w/ cheese	1 item	530	32	11	1	55	1020	40
B.A. Double Bacon Cheese	1 item	800	53	20	2	115	1600	41

Other Items

	Serving	Calories	Total fat (gm)	Saturated fat (gm)	Trans fats (gm)	Cholesterol (mg)	Sodium (mg)	Carbs (gm)
Krystal Chik	1 item	240	11	4	NA	25	640	24
Plain Pup	1 item	170	9	4	NA	25	500	15
Chili Cheese Pup	1 item	210	12	5	NA	40	510	17
Corn Pup	1 item	260	19	8	NA	50	480	19

Side Items

	Serving	Calories	Total fat (gm)	Saturated fat (gm)	Trans fats (gm)	Cholesterol (mg)	Sodium (mg)	Carbs (gm)
French Fries (medium)	4.25 oz.	420	20	8	NA	20	90	53
Chili Cheese Fries	7.5 oz.	540	28	13	NA	45	800	59
Chicken Bites (small)	4 oz.	310	19	8	NA	55	790	16
Chicken Bites Salad w/o dressing	1 salad	290	20	11	NA	65	490	12
Krystal Chili	7.75 oz.	200	7	4	NA	25	1130	22
Lemon Ice Box Pie	1 slice	260	9	2	0	25	180	41
Fried Apple Turnover	1 item	220	10	4	0	<5	300	31

Little Caesars®

14" Round Pizza (medium) 1 of 10 slices

	Serving	Calories	Total fat (gm)	Saturated fat (gm)	Trans fats (gm)	Cholesterol (mg)	Sodium (mg)	Carbs (gm)
Cheese	1 slice	200	7	3	NA	15	320	25
Pepperoni	1 slice	230	8	4	NA	20	430	25
Supreme	1 slice	270	10	5	NA	25	510	26
Meatsa	1 slice	280	13	6	NA	30	630	25
Veggie	1 slice	240	8	4	NA	15	710	27

14" Thin Crust Pizza (medium)

	Serving	Calories	Total fat (gm)	Saturated fat (gm)	Trans fats (gm)	Cholesterol (mg)	Sodium (mg)	Carbs (gm)
Cheese	1 slice	160	7	4	NA	15	210	NA
Pepperoni	1 slice	180	9	5	NA	20	320	NA

14" Deep Dish Pizza (medium)

	Serving	Calories	Total fat (gm)	Saturated fat (gm)	Trans fats (gm)	Cholesterol (mg)	Sodium (mg)	Carbs (gm)
Cheese	1 slice	230	9	4	NA	15	340	38
Pepperoni	1 slice	260	11	5	NA	20	450	38

Pizza by the Slice

	Serving	Calories	Total fat (gm)	Saturated fat (gm)	Trans fats (gm)	Cholesterol (mg)	Sodium (mg)	Carbs (gm)
Cheese	1 slice	330	11	5	NA	25	530	NA
Pepperoni	1 slice	390	14	7	NA	35	750	NA

Little Caesars®
Continued

Deli-Style Cold Items	Serving	Calories	Total fat (gm)	Saturated fat (gm)	Trans fats (gm)	Cholesterol (mg)	Sodium (mg)	Carbs (gm)
Ham & Cheese Sandwich	1 item	640	29	3	NA	50	1540	NA
Italian Sandwich	1 item	800	45	10	NA	90	1950	NA
Veggie Sandwich	1 item	600	28	3	NA	30	980	NA
Other Menu Items								
Baby Pan! Pan!	1 pizza	360	16	7	NA	30	630	33
Chicken Wings	1 item	70	5	2	NA	25	210	1
Crazy Bread	1 item	90	3	1	NA	1	140	15
Cinnamon Crazy Bread	2 item	100	2	1	NA	1	95	NA
Crazy Sauce	4 oz.	45	0	0	NA	0	380	10
Italian Cheese Bread	1 item	130	6	3	NA	10	310	13
Salads (w/o dressing)								
Tossed Salad	1 salad	100	3	1	NA	0	190	NA
Antipasto Salad	1 salad	140	8	2	NA	20	560	NA
Greek Salad	1 salad	120	7	5	NA	25	590	NA
Caesar Salad	1 salad	90	3	1	NA	0	190	NA

Lone Star Steakhouse®

Appetizers	Serving	Calories	Total fat (gm)	Saturated fat (gm)	Trans fats (gm)	Cholesterol (mg)	Sodium (mg)	Carbs (gm)
Chicken Tenders	1 order	378	15	4	NA	152	129	3
Jalapeño Poppers	1 order	420	24	12	NA	60	900	NA
Lone Star Wings	1 order	1759	131	33	NA	335	1470	57
Texas Rose	1 order	953	62	20	NA	108	790	71
Desserts								
Big Brownie Blast	1 order	1390	69	30	NA	144	608	178
Homemade Cobbler	1 order	239	8	1	NA	0	136	43
Homemade Ice Cream	1 order	255	19	12	NA	69	31	NA
Mesquite-Grilled Steaks								
Cajun Ribeye	16 oz.	1248	101	42	NA	304	256	0
Chopped Steak	10 oz.	900	71	29	NA	252	240	0
Delmonico	11 oz.	858	69	29	NA	209	176	0
Five-Star Fillet	9 oz.	738	60	24	NA	180	126	0
New York Strip	14 oz.	1036	80	32	NA	266	210	0
San Antonio Sirloin	12 oz.	768	55	22	NA	228	180	0
T-Bone	20 oz.	1540	124	50	NA	380	280	0
Texas Ribeye	14 oz.	1092	88	36	NA	266	224	0
Other Selections								
Baby Back Ribs	12 oz.	972	80	32	NA	264	252	0

Lone Star Steakhouse® Continued

	Serving	Calories	Total fat (gm)	Saturated fat (gm)	Trans fats (gm)	Cholesterol (mg)	Sodium (mg)	Carbs (gm)
Other Selections continued								
Grilled Chicken	6 oz.	186	2	0	NA	96	108	0
Grilled Pork Chops	16 oz.	1432	100	36	NA	440	316	0
Sweet Bourbon Salmon	6 oz.	240	11	2	NA	96	678	0
Prime Rib								
Prime Rib Slow Roasted	16 oz.	1248	101	42	NA	304	256	0
Salads								
Chicken Caesar Salad	1 order	457	10	5	NA	106	902	31
Dinner Caesar Salad	1 order	158	4	2	NA	5	447	NA
Dinner Salad	1 order	287	19	9	NA	45	381	14
El Paso Salad	1 order	385	23	22	NA	246	707	21
El Paso Salmon	1 order	200	9	2	NA	80	565	NA
El Paso Shrimp	1 order	207	3	1	NA	297	290	23
El Paso Sirloin	1 order	288	21	8	NA	86	68	21
Lettuce Wedge	1 order	507	48	13	NA	22	436	12
Sides								
Baked Potato	1 order	663	18	6	NA	24	1623	114
Baked Sweet Potato	1 order	637	8	5	NA	20	37	137
Sautéed Mushrooms	1 order	115	9	2	NA	0	596	6
Sautéed Onions	1 order	97	7	1	NA	0	495	8
Steamed Vegetables	1 order	71	1	0	NA	0	912	14
Texas Rice	1 order	80	2	1	NA	6	207	12
Soups & Chili								
Black Bean Soup	6 fl. oz.	189	4	1	NA	4	448	NA
Chicken Pot Pie	6 fl. oz.	660	20	10	NA	14	621	NA
Lone Star Chili	6 fl. oz.	228	15	6	NA	53	567	8
Steak Soup	6 fl. oz.	277	18	9	NA	69	324	NA

Fast Food Factoid:
All the information in this guide is of no value unless you chose more GREEN foods and fewer RED foods.

NOTES:
_____
_____
_____
_____

Long John Silver's®

Fish & Seafood	Serving	Calories	Total fat (gm)	Saturated fat (gm)	Trans fats (gm)	Cholesterol (mg)	Sodium (mg)	Carbs (gm)
Alaskan Flounder	1 item	250	11	3	3	35	910	26
Battered Fish	1 item	260	16	4	5	35	790	17
Baked Cod	1 item	120	5	1	0	90	240	1
Battered Shrimp	1 item	45	3	1	1	15	160	3
Buttered Lobster Bites	1 box	250	9	3	4	65	560	27
Giant Shrimp	1 item	80	5	2	2	20	250	NA
Crunchy Shrimp Basket	21 items	380	22	5	5	110	850	NA
Breaded Clams	3 oz.	240	13	2	1	10	1110	29
Popcorn Shrimp	1 box	270	16	4	5	75	570	23
Chicken & Fish								
Chicken Plank	1 item	140	8	2	2	20	480	9
Fish item	1 item	440	20	5	5	35	1120	48
Ultimate Fish item	1 item	500	25	8	5	50	1310	49
Chicken item	1 item	360	15	4	3	25	810	40
Salads								
Shrimp & Seafood Salad	1 salad	260	12	5	2	85	820	22
Chicken Club Salad	1 salad	510	30	9	7	65	1550	35
Dipping Sauces								
Cocktail Sauce	1 oz.	25	0	0	0	0	250	6
Tartar Sauce	1 oz.	100	9	2	0	15	250	4
Sides & Starters								
French Fries (regular)	3 oz.	230	10	3	3	0	350	34
French Fries (large)	5 oz.	390	17	4	5	0	580	56
Hushpuppies	1 item	60	3	1	1	0	200	9
Lobster Stuffed Crab Cake	1 item	170	9	2	0	30	390	16
Cole Slaw	4 oz.	200	15	3	0	20	340	15
Corn Cobbette	1 item	90	3	1	0	0	0	14
Cheesesticks	3 item	140	8	2	2	10	320	12
Rice	4 oz.	180	4	1	0	0	540	34
Crumblies	1 oz.	170	12	3	4	0	420	14
Clam Chowder	8 oz.	220	10	4	1	25	810	19
Desserts								
Chocolate Cream Pie	1 item	310	22	14	2	15	170	24
Pineapple Cream Pie	1 item	290	13	7	2	15	210	39
Pecan Pie	1 item	370	15	3	2	40	190	55

Longhorn Steakhouse®
Does not provide nutrition information.

McDonald's®

	Serving	Calories	Total fat (gm)	Saturated fat (gm)	Trans fats (gm)	Cholesterol (mg)	Sodium (mg)	Carbs (gm)
Breakfast								
Egg McMuffin	1 item	290	11	5	0	235	850	30
Sausage McMuffin	1 item	370	21	9	1	45	790	29
Sausage McMuffin w/ egg	1 item	450	26	10	1	260	930	30
English Muffin	1 item	150	2	1	0	0	260	27
Bacon, Egg & Cheese Biscuit	1 item	440	24	8	5	245	1250	36
Sausage Biscuit w/ egg	1 item	500	32	10	5	250	1080	35
Sausage Biscuit	1 item	410	26	8	5	30	990	33
Biscuit	1 item	240	11	3	5	0	680	32
Bacon, Egg & Cheese McGriddle	1 item	450	21	7	2	245	1260	48
Sausage, Egg & Cheese McGriddle	1 item	560	32	11	2	260	1290	48
Sausage McGriddle	1 item	420	22	7	3	30	990	44
Big Breakfast	1 meal	730	46	14	7	465	1460	49
Deluxe Breakfast	1 meal	1220	60	17	11	480	1900	109
Sausage Burrito	1 item	300	16	6	1	175	760	26
Hotcakes w/o margarine & syrup	1 order	350	9	2	0	20	590	60
Hotcakes & Sausage	1 order	770	33	9	4	50	930	61
Sausage Patty	1.5 oz.	170	15	6	0	30	310	1
Scrambled Eggs	2 eggs	180	11	4	0	435	180	1
Hash Browns	2 oz.	140	8	2	2	0	290	15
Warm Cinnamon Roll	1 roll	420	18	5	5	60	400	NA
Deluxe Warm Cinnamon Roll	1 roll	590	24	7	6	55	660	NA
Items								
Hamburger	1 item	260	9	4	1	30	530	31
Cheeseburger	1 item	310	12	6	1	40	740	33
Double Cheeseburger	1 item	460	23	11	2	80	1140	34
Quarter Pounder	1 item	420	18	7	1	70	730	37
Quarter Pounder w/ cheese	1 item	510	25	12	2	95	1150	40
Big Mac	1 item	560	30	10	2	80	1010	45
Big 'n Tasty	1 item	520	29	9	2	80	730	37
Big 'n Tasty w/ cheese	1 item	570	33	11	2	90	960	38
Fillet-O-Fish	1 item	400	18	4	1	40	640	38
Chicken McGrill	1 item	400	16	3	0	70	1010	51
Crispy Chicken	1 item	500	23	4	2	50	1090	61
Hot 'n Spicy Chicken	1 item	440	24	5	1	45	920	NA
McChicken	1 item	420	22	5	1	45	760	40
Side Items & Sauces								
French Fries (small)	2.5 oz.	230	11	2	3	0	140	30
French Fries (medium)	4 oz.	350	16	3	4	0	220	47

McDonald's®
Continued

Side Items & Sauces continued

	Serving	Calories	Total fat (gm)	Saturated fat (gm)	Trans fats (gm)	Cholesterol (mg)	Sodium (mg)	Carbs (gm)
Chicken McNuggets	4 pieces	170	10	2	1	25	450	10
Chicken McNuggets	6 pieces	250	15	3	2	35	670	15
Barbeque Sauce	1 oz.	45	0	0	0	0	260	12
Honey	.5 oz.	50	0	0	0	0	0	12
Hot Mustard Sauce	1 oz.	50	2	0	0	0	260	9
Snack wrap w/ Crispy Chicken	1 item	330	16	5	1	30	780	32
Snack Wrap w/ Grilled Chicken	1 item	270	10	4	0	45	830	26
Sweet 'n Sour Sauce	1 oz.	50	0	0	0	0	160	12
Chicken Selects Breast Strips	3 pieces	380	20	4	3	55	930	28
Chicken Selects Breast Strips	5 pieces	630	33	6	5	90	1550	46
Spicy Buffalo Sauce	1.5 oz.	60	6	1	0	0	910	1
Creamy Ranch Sauce	1.5 oz.	200	21	4	0	10	300	2
Tangy Honey Mustard Sauce	1.5 oz.	70	2	0	0	0	160	13

Salads (w/o dressing)

	Serving	Calories	Total fat (gm)	Saturated fat (gm)	Trans fats (gm)	Cholesterol (mg)	Sodium (mg)	Carbs (gm)
Bacon Ranch w/o chicken	1 salad	130	7	4	0	25	290	10
Bacon Ranch w/ grilled chicken	1 salad	240	9	4	0	85	940	12
Bacon Ranch w/ crispy chicken	1 salad	340	16	5	2	65	1030	23
Caesar Salad	1 salad	90	4	3	0	10	170	9
Caesar Salad w/ grilled chicken	1 salad	200	6	3	0	70	830	12
Caesar Salad w/ crispy chicken	1 salad	300	14	5	2	50	910	22
California Cobb Salad	1 salad	150	9	4	0	85	400	NA
California Cobb Salad w/ grilled chicken	1 salad	260	11	5	0	145	1060	NA
California Cobb Salad w/ crispy chicken	1 salad	360	18	6	2	125	1140	NA
Fruit & Walnut Salad w/ yogurt	1 salad	210	8	1.5	0	5	60	31
Southwest Salad w/ Grilled Chicken	1 salad	320	9	3	0	70	970	30
Southwest Salad w/ Crispy Chicken	1 salad	40	16	4	2	50	1110	41
Southwest Salad (no chicken)	1 salad	140	4	2	0	10	150	20
Asian Salad w/ Grilled Chicken	1 salad	300	10	1	0	65	890	23
Asian Salad w/ Crispy Chicken	1 salad	380	17	3	2	45	1030	33
Asian Salad (no chicken)	1 salad	150	7	1	0	0	35	15
Side Salad	1 salad	20	0	0	0	0	10	4

Desserts

	Serving	Calories	Total fat (gm)	Saturated fat (gm)	Trans fats (gm)	Cholesterol (mg)	Sodium (mg)	Carbs (gm)
Fruit 'n Yogurt Parfait	1 item	160	2	1	0	5	85	31
Fruit 'n Yogurt Parfait w/o granola	1 item	130	2	1	0	5	55	25
Apple Dippers	2.5 oz.	35	0	0	0	0	0	8
Low-Fat Caramel Dip	.75 oz.	70	1	1	0	5	35	15
Baked Apple Pie	1 item	250	11	3	5	0	150	36

Nathan's Famous®

	Serving	Calories	Total fat (gm)	Saturated fat (gm)	Trans fats (gm)	Cholesterol (mg)	Sodium (mg)	Carbs (gm)
Hot Dogs								
Hot Dog	1 item	309	20	8	NA	35	684	NA
Hot Dog Nuggets	6 item	351	28	4	NA	20	400	NA
Burgers								
Nathan's ¼ lb. Hamburger	1 item	537	30	12	NA	90	813	NA
Nathan's ¼ lb. Cheeseburger	1 item	850	61	21	NA	136	1239	NA
Super Burger	1 item	864	62	21	NA	136	1245	NA
Bacon Cheeseburger	1 item	707	44	20	NA	128	1340	NA
Cheesesteaks								
Original Cheesesteak	1 item	741	43	19	NA	124	1239	NA
Cheesesteak Supreme	1 item	786	43	19	NA	124	1525	NA
Chicken Cheesesteak	1 item	565	19	10	NA	81	1786	NA
Seafood								
Fish item	1 item	469	20	4	NA	34	750	NA
Fish 'n Chips	1 meal	1538	101	17	NA	111	2152	NA
Shrimp 'n Chips	1 meal	2051	124	13	NA	222	3433	NA
Seafood Sampler	1 meal	3379	270	29	NA	156	3553	NA
Chicken								
Grilled Chicken item	1 item	523	29	5	NA	67	1179	NA
Chicken Tender item	1 item	725	47	7	NA	65	1007	NA
Chicken Tender Pita	1 item	610	38	5	NA	645	1009	NA
Chicken Breast Platter	1 meal	943	54	7	NA	84	978	NA
Chicken Tender Platter	1 meal	1301	83	10	NA	105	1059	NA
Chicken Tenders	3 pieces	512	37	5	NA	30	900	NA
Side Items								
French Fries (regular)	9.75 oz.	546	38	4	NA	0	200	NA
French Fries (large)	13.5 oz.	758	52	5	NA	0	278	NA
Onion Rings (small)	5.75 oz.	558	44	6	NA	0	576	NA
Cole Slaw	5 oz.	213	8	1	NA	7	326	NA
Corn Muffin	1 item	163	6	1	NA	0	244	NA
Hush Puppy	2 item	277	10	2	NA	5	967	NA

Fast Food Factoid:

Nathan's Famous has the number one fast food in America…if you are counting calories. The Seafood Sampler has 3,379 calories! It also has 270 grams of fat. You should come home with leftovers for several days.

Noble Roman's®

14" Traditional Pizza

	Serving	Calories	Total fat (gm)	Saturated fat (gm)	Trans fats (gm)	Cholesterol (mg)	Sodium (mg)	Carbs (gm)
Cheese	1 slice	191	7	3	NA	15	460	24
Pepperoni	1 slice	224	10	5	NA	23	580	24
Sausage	1 slice	277	15	6	NA	28	653	24
The Works	1 slice	302	16	7	NA	35	768	26
Items								
Baked Ham & Cheese	1 item	787	54	20	NA	94	2541	43
Baked Italian Roast Beef	1 item	750	49	17	NA	112	2636	37
Baked Stromboli	1 item	1012	72	28	NA	133	2985	50
Side Items								
Hot Wings	6 item	360	28	7	NA	111	519	3
BBQ Wings	6 item	360	22	6	NA	100	1028	15
Breadsticks w/ cheese	3 item	410	12	4	NA	15	1050	59
Calzone Pizza Stuffer	1 item	420	18	6	NA	35	1040	48

Fast Food Factoid:

McDonald's restaurants announced in 2002 that they were going to introduce a new cooking oil into all of its restaurants. The oil was supposed to have half the amount of trans fats as their previous frying oil. Two years later, they hadn't changed anything. A group in California sued. McDonald's lost and has since donated $7 million to the American Heart Association, to be used to educate the public about the dangers of eating foods fried in trans fats. For more information go to www.bantransfats.com

---

O'Charley's®

Appetizers

	Serving	Calories	Total fat (gm)	Saturated fat (gm)	Trans fats (gm)	Cholesterol (mg)	Sodium (mg)	Carbs (gm)
Spinach & Artichoke Dip	½ order	661	41	11	NA	12	1222	NA
Chicken Quesadilla	1 item	1133	81	34	NA	162	2017	NA
Chicken Tenders Appetizer	½ order	580	15	3	NA	57	2644	NA
Three Cheese Shrimp Dip	½ order	625	38	12	NA	100	1104	NA
Buffalo Tenders	½ order	715	22	5	NA	57	3056	NA
Chipotle Tenders	½ order	742	11	3	NA	54	3231	NA
Onion Tanglers	½ order	420	29	5	NA	0	450	NA
Chips & Salsa	½ order	455	23	4	NA	0	784	NA
Loaded Potato Skins	½ order	563	40	24	NA	120	2218	NA
Fried Cheese Wedges	½ order	265	15	9	NA	50	581	NA

O'Charley's®
Continued

Brunch	Serving	Calories	Total fat (gm)	Saturated fat (gm)	Trans fats (gm)	Cholesterol (mg)	Sodium (mg)	Carbs (gm)
Ultimate Omelette w/ fries & bread	1 meal	970	66	20	NA	798	1498	NA
Ham & Cheese Omelette w/ fries & bread	1 meal	949	67	21	NA	804	1640	NA
Spanish Omelette w/ fries & bread	1 meal	956	70	23	NA	791	1262	NA
Steak & Eggs	1 order	975	54	21	NA	672	824	NA
Bavarian Waffles w/ syrup	1 order	831	24	5	NA	0	1572	NA
Waffles w/ strawberries	1 order	971	33	10	NA	29	1622	NA
Pecan Waffles w/ syrup	1 order	1225	63	13	NA	29	1621	NA
Fried Eggs	2 eggs	274	23	6	NA	501	265	NA
Bacon	3 slices	109	9	3	NA	16	303	NA
Sausage	2 links	96	8	3	NA	22	336	NA
Brunch Potatoes	1 order	198	10	2	NA	0	222	NA
Soups & Salads								
Loaded Potato Soup	1 cup	212	11	3	NA	14	1385	NA
Vegetable Steamer w/ reduced-fat ranch dressing	1 salad	725	36	5	NA	0	2710	NA
House Salad w/o dressing	1 salad	245	14	7	NA	39	1232	NA
Caesar Salad	1 salad	464	38	11	NA	30	584	NA
Chicken Caesar Salad	1 salad	620	40	11	NA	112	678	NA
Salmon Caesar Salad	1 salad	773	52	13	NA	151	680	NA
Black & Blue Caesar Salad	1 salad	1008	66	24	NA	220	2065	NA
Items								
Roast Beef Stack	1 item	930	64	22	NA	161	639	NA
Chicken item	1 item	470	21	5	NA	91	594	NA
Buffalo Chicken item	1 item	559	14	3	NA	83	1763	NA
Bacon & Cheese Chicken Sandwich	1 item	760	45	17	NA	155	1420	NA
Cajun Chicken item	1 item	483	21	5	NA	91	1542	NA
Half-Pound Cheeseburger	1 item	1129	73	28	NA	234	1107	NA
Southern Fried BLT	1 item	848	21	7	NA	88	3646	NA
Fisherman's TLC w/ sauce	1 item	672	25	7	NA	259	1732	NA
Steaks (entrée only unless otherwise noted)								
Ribeye Steak	1 order	903	71	32	NA	228	547	NA
Petite Sirloin	7 oz.	317	13	6	NA	134	456	NA
Filet Mignon	1 order	756	53	22	NA	219	479	NA
Chopped Steak on Smashed Potatoes	1 order	1427	97	32	NA	263	1201	NA
Steak Tips Monterey on Rice	1 order	1143	82	27	NA	169	1333	NA
Steak & Fried Shrimp Combo	1 order	620	28	8	NA	347	1023	NA

	Serving	Calories	Total fat (gm)	Saturated fat (gm)	Trans fats (gm)	Cholesterol (mg)	Sodium (mg)	Carbs (gm)
Steaks (entrée only unless otherwise noted) continued								
Steak & Grilled Shrimp Combo	1 order	570	19	7	NA	177	1120	NA
Prime Rib	8 oz.	932	80	36	NA	191	147	NA
Chicken (entrée only unless otherwise noted)								
Chicken Tenders Dinner w/ sauce	6 items	1359	34	7	NA	137	6320	NA
Chicken Florentine on Linguini Alfredo w/ vegetable medley	1 meal	960	38	12	NA	165	1483	NA
Chicken Teriyaki on Rice Pilaf w/ vegetable medley	1 meal	689	17	3	NA	132	3052	NA
Grilled Chicken on Potatoes w/ vegetable medley	1 meal	547	18	4	NA	139	1140	NA
Chicken Parmesan on Linguini w/ vegetable medley	1 meal	841	27	10	NA	116	1894	NA
Seafood (entrée only unless otherwise noted)								
Fried Shrimp Platter (shrimp only)	8 item	549	28	5	NA	401	780	NA
Grilled Shrimp on Rice w/ cocktail sauce	1 order	387	18	3	NA	85	1511	NA
Grilled Salmon	6 oz.	532	32	6	NA	167	635	NA
Chipotle Salmon	6 oz.	594	32	6	NA	167	871	NA
Blackened Trout	8 oz.	424	24	5	NA	134	664	NA
Grilled Tuna w/ sauce	9 oz.	410	16	2	NA	115	926	NA
Side Items								
Baked Potato (plain)	1 item	200	1	1	NA	0	15	NA
Smashed Potatoes	1 order	340	14	5	NA	20	1098	NA
French Fries	1 order	402	21	5	NA	0	449	NA
Rice Pilaf	1 order	221	6	1	NA	0	623	NA
Vegetable Medley	1 order	135	8	1	NA	0	421	NA
Cole Slaw	1 order	215	14	2	NA	5	566	NA
Roll	1 roll	162	2	0	NA	0	112	NA

Fast Food Factoid:

Some day healthy people are going to feel really stupid, lying in hospital beds dying of nothing.

—Author Unknown

Old Country Buffet®

	Serving	Calories	Total fat (gm)	Saturated fat (gm)	Trans fats (gm)	Cholesterol (mg)	Sodium (mg)	Carbs (gm)
Breakfast								
Bacon	3 slices	90	8	3	NA	30	435	NA
Sausage Link	1 item	100	10	4	NA	30	170	NA
Poached Egg	2 oz	70	5	2	NA	3	150	NA
Eggs Benedict	5 oz	250	15	4	NA	225	840	NA
Scrambled Eggs	2.25 oz.	130	11	3	NA	250	80	0
Denver Scrambled Eggs	2.75 oz.	140	11	3	NA	240	220	NA
Breakfast Quiche	3.75 oz.	220	15	5	NA	120	450	NA
French Toast	1 item	170	8	2	NA	100	190	24
Pancake	1 item	120	4	1	NA	0	280	19
Waffle	1 item	120	3	1	NA	0	440	19
Breakfast Sides								
Biscuit	1 item	180	7	2	NA	0	450	24
Corn Muffin	1 item	230	6	2	NA	0	480	NA
English Muffin	1 item	60	1	0	NA	0	130	13
Hash Browns	3 oz.	110	6	1	NA	0	140	NA
Grits	4 oz.	70	0	0	NA	0	140	NA
Oatmeal	4 oz.	70	1	0	NA	0	120	NA
Breakfast Rolls								
Glazed Donut	1 item	130	7	2	NA	0	40	NA
Cinnamon Sugar Donut Holes	3 items	150	9	2	NA	0	225	5
Caramel Roll	1 roll	140	5	1	NA	0	110	NA
Glazed Cinnamon Roll	1 roll	150	2	1	NA	0	105	NA
Salad & Fruit Bar								
Caesar Salad	1 cup	80	6	1	NA	10	130	5
Carrot & Raisin Salad	3.5 oz.	140	8	1	NA	10	110	18
Chicken Pasta Salad	3.5 oz.	230	18	3	NA	45	290	11
Creamy Coleslaw	3.5 oz.	160	13	2	NA	10	270	NA
Creamy Pea Salad	3.5 oz.	160	11	4	NA	25	170	11
Cucumber Tomato Salad	3.5 oz.	30	1	0	NA	0	390	6
Greek Salad	2.5 oz.	120	8	2	NA	5	220	11
Marinated Vegetables	3.5 oz.	60	4	1	NA	0	140	6
Potato Salad	2.5 oz.	110	5	1	NA	20	200	14
Seafood Salad	4 oz.	310	26	4	NA	40	400	16
Three Bean Salad	3.5 oz.	90	5	1	NA	0	480	12
Waldorf Salad	3 oz.	110	7	1	NA	5	25	12
Soups								
Chicken Noodle	4 oz.	70	2	1	NA	30	360	7
Chicken Rice	4 oz.	70	2	1	NA	25	360	8
Chili Bean	4 oz.	100	4	1	NA	20	370	9

Old Country Buffet® Continued

Soups continued

	Serving	Calories	Total fat (gm)	Saturated fat (gm)	Trans fats (gm)	Cholesterol (mg)	Sodium (mg)	Carbs (gm)
Cream of Broccoli	4 oz.	80	7	4	NA	0	250	5
Navy Bean w/ ham	4 oz.	50	1	0	NA	0	410	10
Dinner Entrées								
Beef BBQ Ribs	5 oz.	300	23	9	NA	60	350	7
Beef Liver & Onions	3 oz.	80	3	1	NA	160	190	4
Carved Ham	3 oz.	140	9	3	NA	45	970	0
Carved Peppered Pork Loin	3 oz.	160	8	4	NA	70	55	0
Carved Roast Beef	3 oz.	230	15	7	NA	70	55	0
Carved Roast Turkey	3 oz.	170	8	3	NA	70	60	0
Chicken & Dumplings	5 oz.	190	7	2	NA	20	710	24
Chicken Cacciatore	5 oz.	220	11	3	NA	95	320	3
Fried Chicken Breast	1 item	310	16	5	NA	150	470	3
Fried Chicken Drumstick	1 item	90	6	2	NA	50	110	2
Fried Chicken Thigh	1 item	210	14	4	NA	115	250	4
Baked Chicken Breast	1 item	280	12	4	NA	125	230	0
Baked Chicken Drumstick	1 item	90	6	2	NA	35	100	0
Baked Chicken Thigh	1 item	160	11	3	NA	60	180	0
Crustless Chicken Pot Pie	5 oz.	230	12	3	NA	95	370	NA
Cheese Pizza	1 slice	80	4	2	NA	10	210	NA
Three-Cheese Deep Dish Pizza	1 slice	160	10	4	NA	20	430	NA
Pepperoni & Sausage Deep Dish Pizza	1 slice	200	13	5	NA	30	540	NA
Fish Patties	2.5 oz.	160	9	2	NA	25	430	13
Baked Fish	3 oz.	120	4	1	NA	70	240	NA
Fried Fish	1.25 oz.	80	4	1	NA	10	130	9
Italian Sausage w/ vegetables	3 oz.	160	13	5	NA	30	410	NA
Macaroni & Cheese	3.5 oz.	150	3	2	NA	5	610	NA
Meatloaf	3.25 oz.	220	12	5	NA	80	270	NA
Pot Roast w/ gravy	4 oz.	210	16	7	NA	65	90	NA
Vegetables for Pot Roast & Gravy	4 oz.	50	1	0	NA	0	60	NA
Smoked Sausage	1 link	190	17	8	NA	25	460	2
Sauerkraut	1 oz.	5	0	0	NA	0	110	1
Spaghetti	3 oz.	90	1	0	NA	0	90	NA
Italian Meatballs w/ sauce	1 item	50	3	1	NA	15	110	NA
Meat Sauce	2 oz.	70	3	1	NA	15	360	NA
Marinara Sauce	2 oz.	30	1	0	NA	0	260	NA
Dinner Side Items								
Breadstick	1 item	140	5	1	NA	0	260	21
Cornbread (plain)	1 item	140	4	1	NA	0	270	NA
Savory Yeast Dinner Roll	1 roll	120	4	1	NA	0	200	NA

Old Country Buffet® Continued

Dinner Side Items continued

	Serving	Calories	Total fat (gm)	Saturated fat (gm)	Trans fats (gm)	Cholesterol (mg)	Sodium (mg)	Carbs (gm)
Baked Beans	4 oz.	120	1	0	NA	0	530	29
Bread Dressing	3.5 oz.	130	4	1	NA	10	460	21
Steamed Carrots	3 oz.	40	0	0	NA	0	45	9
Steamed Corn	3 oz.	100	1	0	NA	0	210	21
Corn on the Cob	1 item	100	3	1	NA	0	0	16
Creamy Cheese Sauce	2 oz.	50	2	1	NA	2	630	9
French Fries	2 oz.	190	9	2	NA	0	380	24
Fried Rice w/ ham	3.5 oz.	170	6	2	NA	75	640	23
Green Bean Casserole	4 oz.	60	3	1	NA	0	210	9
Green Beans	3 oz.	15	0	0	NA	0	250	3
Herbed Broccoli	3 oz.	40	2	1	NA	0	55	NA
Italian-Style Green Beans w/ bacon	3 oz.	60	4	1	NA	0	280	NA
Montreal Vegetable Medley	3 oz.	40	4	1	NA	0	110	3
Baked Potato	1 item	160	0	0	NA	0	10	39
Cowboy Grilled Potatoes	4 oz.	110	5	1	NA	0	420	NA
Mashed Potatoes	5 oz.	150	3	1	NA	0	710	NA
Beef Gravy	2 oz.	30	2	1	NA	4	210	NA
Chicken Gravy	2 oz.	30	1	0	NA	0	250	NA
Country Gravy	2 oz.	120	8	3	NA	0	590	NA
Red Potatoes	4 oz.	100	3	1	NA	0	10	18
Red Beans w/ ham	3 oz.	90	1	0	NA	0	440	18
Scalloped Potatoes w/ ham	6 oz.	120	7	3	NA	20	630	NA
Vegetable Stir-Fry	3 oz.	25	1	0	NA	0	180	6
Wild Rice Vegetable Pilaf	3.5 oz.	90	1	0	NA	0	370	17
Candied Yams	4.5 oz.	140	2	0	NA	0	55	30

Olive Garden®
Does not provide nutrition information.

Outback Steakhouse®
Does not provide nutrition information.

Panda Express®

	Serving	Calories	Total fat (gm)	Saturated fat (gm)	Trans fats (gm)	Cholesterol (mg)	Sodium (mg)	Carbs (gm)
Appetizers								
Fried Shrimp	6 item	260	12	3	0	65	730	NA
Veggie Spring Roll	1 roll	80	3	0	0	0	270	11
Chicken Egg Roll	1 roll	190	8	2	0	25	450	17
Chicken Potsticker	3 pieces	220	12	2	0	0	360	25
Cream Cheese Rangoon	3 pieces	190	8	5	0	35	180	24
Chicken Entrées								
Black Pepper Chicken	5.5 oz.	180	10	2	0	40	630	11
Orange Flavored Chicken	5.5 oz.	480	21	5	0	80	820	42
Chicken w/ mushrooms	5.5 oz.	130	7	2	0	50	590	8
Chicken w/ string beans	5.5 oz.	170	8	2	0	30	560	NA
Kung Pao Chicken	5.5 oz.	240	15	3	0	65	540	12
Spicy Chicken w/ peanuts	5.5 oz.	200	7	2	0	70	800	NA
Mandarin Chicken	5.5 oz.	250	9	3	0	125	960	NA
Mushroom Chicken	5.5 oz.	130	6	2	0	45	520	NA
Potato Chicken	5.5 oz.	200	10	2	0	55	990	21
Chicken w/ potato	5.5 oz.	220	11	2	0	55	910	NA
String Bean Chicken Breast	5.5 oz.	160	8	2	0	25	550	10
Sweet & Sour Chicken	4 oz.	310	14	3	0	50	330	NA
Shrimp								
Tangy Shrimp	5.5 oz.	150	5	1	0	85	550	16
Kung Pao Shrimp	5.5 oz.	240	14	2	0	95	640	14
Crispy Shrimp	6 pieces	260	13	3	0	60	810	26
Beef & Pork Entrées								
Beef w/ broccoli	5.5 oz.	150	8	2	0	15	730	11
Beef w/ string beans	5.5 oz.	170	9	2	0	20	640	NA
Mongolian Beef	5.5 oz.	180	11	2	0	25	800	15
Sweet & Sour Pork	4 oz.	410	30	7	0	55	350	35
BBQ Pork	4 ½ oz	350	19	7	0	85	970	15
Vegetables & Tofu								
Eggplant & Tofu in Garlic Sauce	5.5 oz.	180	10	2	0	0	690	20
Mixed Vegetables	5.5 oz.	70	3	1	0	0	420	8
String Beans w/ fried tofu	5.5 oz.	18	11	2	0	0	650	NA
Rice & Noodles								
Vegetable Fried Rice	8 oz.	390	12	3	0	85	740	67
Steamed Rice	8 oz.	330	1	0	0	0	20	81
Vegetable Chow Mein	8 oz.	330	11	2	0	0	810	59
Soup								
Hot & Sour Soup	12 oz	110	4	1	0	85	1370	14
Egg Flower Soup	12 oz	88	2	0	0	55	895	16

Panera Bread®

	Serving	Calories	Total fat (gm)	Saturated fat (gm)	Trans fats (gm)	Cholesterol (mg)	Sodium (mg)	Carbs (gm)
Breads								
Artisan Three Cheese	2 oz.	120	2	1	0	5	270	24
Asiago Cheese Focaccia	2 oz.	150	6	2	0	5	300	21
Basil Pesto Focaccia	2 oz.	150	6	2	0	5	300	22
Ciabatta	6 oz.	430	10	2	0	0	990	82
Honey Wheat Bread	2 oz.	140	3	1	0	0	260	30
Nine-Grain Bread	2 oz.	150	3	1	0	0	270	NA
Rosemary & Onion Focaccia	2 oz.	140	5	1	0	5	280	22
Rye Bread	2 oz.	140	3	1	0	0	290	25
Sourdough Roll	2.5 oz.	160	0	0	0	0	340	38
Tomato Basil Bread	2 oz.	130	1	0	0	0	350	27
Country	2 oz.	130	0	0	0	0	310	27
French	2 oz.	140	0	0	0	0	370	28
Sesame Smolina	2 oz.	130	1	0	0	0	350	27
Three Cheese	2 oz.	140	2	1	0	5	300	24
Three Seed	2 oz.	140	3	0	0	0	290	25
Whole Grain Baguette	2 oz.	140	1	0	0	0	330	28
Sourdough	2 oz.	150	0	0	0	0	320	30
Sunflower	2 oz.	180	6	0	0	0	280	26
Bagels								
Plain	1 item	280	1	0	0	0	450	61
Lower Carb Plain	1 item	200	2	1	0	0	460	NA
Asiago Cheese	1 item	330	5	3	0	15	480	60
Lower Carb Asiago	1 item	240	9	5	0	20	500	NA
Blueberry	1 item	320	2	0	0	0	490	69
Dutch Apple & Raisin	1 item	340	3	0	0	0	410	78
Everything	1 item	290	2	0	0	0	540	60
French Toast	1 item	340	5	1	0	0	610	73
Nine-Grain	1 item	290	1	0	0	0	390	NA
Pumpkin Spice	1 item	360	2	0	0	0	670	NA
Sesame	1 item	310	3	0	0	0	460	58
Cinnamon Crunch	1 item	410	8	6	0	0	490	75
Mochachip Swirl	1 item	380	4	2	0	0	480	74
Pink Ribbon	1 item	400	6	4	0	0	490	75
Whole Grain	1 item	340	3	1	0	0	410	66
Reduced-Fat Cream Cheese Spread								
Hazelnut	2 oz.	150	11	7	0.5	35	210	6
Honey Walnut	2 oz.	150	11	7	0	30	200	10
Mocha	2 oz.	160	11	7	0	30	180	NA
Plain	2 oz.	130	12	8	0	35	230	2

Panera Bread®
Continued

Reduced-Fat Cream Cheese Spread continued

	Serving	Calories	Total fat (gm)	Saturated fat (gm)	Trans fats (gm)	Cholesterol (mg)	Sodium (mg)	Carbs (gm)
Raspberry	2 oz.	120	10	7	0.5	30	200	8
Sun-Dried Tomato	2 oz.	140	11	7	0.5	35	220	4
Veggie	2 oz.	130	11	7	0.5	35	230	3

Sandwiches

	Serving	Calories	Total fat (gm)	Saturated fat (gm)	Trans fats (gm)	Cholesterol (mg)	Sodium (mg)	Carbs (gm)
Smokehouse Turkey Panini on Artisan Three-Cheese	1 item	670	23	10	0.5	50	2320	37
Turkey Artichoke Panini on Basil Pesto Focaccia	1 item	810	38	11	0.5	25	2470	88
Frontega Chicken Panini on Rosemary & Onion Focaccia	1 item	860	42	12	0.5	110	2260	78
Smoked Turkey Breast on Sourdough	1 item	440	15	2	0	10	1950	76
Tuscan Chicken on Rosemary & Onion Focaccia	1 item	950	57	10	NA	80	2140	NA
Sierra Turkey on Asiago Cheese	1 item	950	55	13	0.5	40	2360	80
Bacon Turkey Bravo on Tomato Basil	1 item	770	28	9	0	45	2850	83
Garden Veggie on Ciabatta	1 item	570	23	7	NA	15	1490	NA
Italian Combo on Ciabatta	1 item	1050	54	18	0	165	3570	91
Smoked Turkey Breast on Artisan Country	1 item	590	16	2	0	10	2320	77
Chicken Salad on Nine Grain	1 item	640	29	5	0	90	1340	71
Tuna Salad on Honey Wheat	1 item	720	43	6	0	65	1570	51
Smoked Ham & Swiss on Rye	1 item	650	34	11	1	110	2350	52

Salads

	Serving	Calories	Total fat (gm)	Saturated fat (gm)	Trans fats (gm)	Cholesterol (mg)	Sodium (mg)	Carbs (gm)
Asian Sesame Chicken Salad w/ Asian vinaigrette	1 salad	330	17	2	NA	65	1170	31
Caesar Salad w/ caesar dressing	1 salad	390	26	8	NA	110	750	25
Grilled Caesar Chicken Salad w/ caesar dressing	1 salad	500	33	8	NA	125	1530	26
Fandango Salad w/ raspberry dressing	1 salad	400	28	7	NA	25	480	NA
Greek Salad w/ Greek dressing	1 salad	520	48	10	NA	20	1560	17
Classic Café Salad w/ balsamic vinaigrette	1 salad	390	37	5	NA	0	350	19
Fuji Apple Chicken	1 salad	290	15	4	0	45	510	38
Grilled Salmon	1 salad	170	7	1	0	25	410	32
Orchard Harvest	1 salad	420	24	8	0	25	690	30
Strawberry Poppyseed & Chicken	1 salad	310	4	1	0	65	530	35
Tomato & Fresh Mozzarella Salad w/ dressing	1 salad	790	55	21	NA	85	790	NA

Soups

	Serving	Calories	Total fat (gm)	Saturated fat (gm)	Trans fats (gm)	Cholesterol (mg)	Sodium (mg)	Carbs (gm)
Asparagus & Chicken Florentine	8 oz.	230	16	9	NA	50	870	NA
Boston Clam Chowder	8 oz.	210	11	6	0.5	40	990	11

Panera Bread®
Continued
Soups continued

	Serving	Calories	Total fat (gm)	Saturated fat (gm)	Trans fats (gm)	Cholesterol (mg)	Sodium (mg)	Carbs (gm)
Broccoli Cheddar	8 oz.	230	16	9	0	45	1000	13
Cream of Chicken & Wild Rice	8 oz.	200	12	6	0	35	970	19
Low-Fat Chicken Noodle	8 oz.	100	2	0	0	15	1080	15
Low-Fat Vegetarian Tomato Basil	8 oz.	110	3	0	0	0	910	NA
Low-Fat Vegetarian Black Bean	8 oz.	160	1	0	0	0	820	31
Low-Fat Vegetarian Garden Vegetable	8 oz.	90	1	0	0	0	860	17
Baked Potato	8 oz.	230	14	7	0	35	670	21
French Onion	8 oz.	80	3	2	0	10	1560	23
Low-Fat Chicken Noodle	8 oz.	100	2	0	0	15	1080	15
Parisian Chicken	8.75 oz	170	11	5	0	30	750	13
Vegetarian Fiesta Con Queso	8.75 oz	250	16	10	0	45	950	18

Papa John's®
14" Original Crust Pizza (large) 1 of 8 slices

	Serving	Calories	Total fat (gm)	Saturated fat (gm)	Trans fats (gm)	Cholesterol (mg)	Sodium (mg)	Carbs (gm)
Cheese	1 slice	300	11	4	0	20	770	39
Pepperoni	1 slice	330	14	5	0	25	860	39
Sausage	1 slice	360	18	5	0	25	910	37
The Meats w/o beef	1 slice	350	16	5	0	30	950	38
Garden Fresh	1 slice	270	9	3	0	10	680	40
The Works	1 slice	360	13	7	0	30	990	39
Grilled Chicken Alfredo	1 slice	300	10	4	0	30	720	36
BBQ Chicken & Bacon	1 slice	330	11	3	0	30	960	44
Hawaiian BBQ Chicken	1 slice	340	11	3	0	30	960	46
Spicy Italian	1 slice	310	11	2	0	35	1020	39
Spinach Alfredo Chicken Tomato	1 slice	300	11	4	0	25	670	37
Spinach Alfredo	1 slice	280	11	5	0	20	630	36
Grilled Chicken Club	1 slice	320	12	4	0	30	820	NA
Italian Meats Trio	1 slice	340	11	7	0	30	1030	38

14" Thin Crust Pizza (large) 1 of 8 slices

	Serving	Calories	Total fat (gm)	Saturated fat (gm)	Trans fats (gm)	Cholesterol (mg)	Sodium (mg)	Carbs (gm)
Cheese	1 slice	260	14	4	0	20	550	22
Pepperoni	1 slice	280	16	5	0	25	640	23
Sausage	1 slice	310	20	6	0	25	690	26
The Meats w/o beef	1 slice	300	18	5	0	30	730	23
Garden Fresh	1 slice	230	11	3	0	10	460	23
The Works	1 slice	310	15	7	0	30	780	24
Grilled Chicken Alfredo	1 slice	250	13	4	0	30	500	20
BBQ Chicken w/ bacon	1 slice	280	13	4	0	30	740	29

Papa John's®
Continued

14" Thin Crust Pizza (large) 1 of 8 slices continued

	Serving	Calories	Total fat (gm)	Saturated fat (gm)	Trans fats (gm)	Cholesterol (mg)	Sodium (mg)	Carbs (gm)
Hawaiian BBQ Chicken	1 slice	290	13	4	0	30	740	31
Spicy Italian	1 slice	260	14	2	0	35	800	24
Spinach Alfredo Chicken Tomato	1 slice	250	13	5	0	25	450	21
Spinach Alfredo	1 slice	220	13	5	0	20	370	19
Grilled Chicken Club	1 slice	270	14	4	0	30	600	NA
Italian Meats Trio	1 slice	280	12	7	0	30	820	22

Sides

	Serving	Calories	Total fat (gm)	Saturated fat (gm)	Trans fats (gm)	Cholesterol (mg)	Sodium (mg)	Carbs (gm)
Breadstick	1 Stick	140	2	0	0	0	260	26
Cheesesticks	2 Sticks	370	16	5	0	25	830	42
Garlic Parmesan Breadsticks	1 Stick	170	6	1	0	0	370	26
Chicken Strips	2 Strips	160	8	2	0	25	350	10
Papas Spicey Buffalo Wings	2 Wings	160	11	4	0	90	680	1
Apple Twist Sweetreat	1/2 Pie	350	9	4	0	0	550	54
Cinna Swirl Sweetreat	1/2 Pie	390	14	5	0	0	580	53
Very Berry Sweetreat	1/2 Pie	400	9	4	0	0	570	67

Perkins Restaurant and Bakery®
Does not provide nutrition information.

P. F. Chang's®
Provides very limited nutritional information.

Appetizers

	Serving	Calories	Total fat (gm)	Saturated fat (gm)	Trans fats (gm)	Cholesterol (mg)	Sodium (mg)	Carbs (gm)
Chang's Chicken in Lettuce Wraps	1 order	630	8	2	NA	NA	NA	68
Crab Wontons	1 order	520	26	8	NA	NA	NA	52
Harvest Spring Rolls	1 order	640	17	2	NA	NA	NA	46
Pan-Fried Peking Dumplings	1 item	420	22	7	NA	NA	NA	31
Pan-Fried Shrimp Dumplings	1 item	360	17	2	NA	NA	NA	26
Pan-Fried Vegetable Dumplings	1 item	340	12	1	NA	NA	NA	53
Shanghai Street Dumplings	1 order	860	46	4	NA	NA	NA	NA
Chang's Spare Ribs	1 order	1280	79	20	NA	NA	NA	47
Chang's Vegetarian Lettuce Wraps	1 order	420	5	0	NA	NA	NA	70
Northern Style Spare Ribs	1 order	730	55	12	NA	NA	NA	6
Salt & Pepper Calamari	1 order	770	50	4	NA	NA	NA	28
Seared Ahi Tuna	1 order	260	6	1	NA	NA	NA	21

Soups

	Serving	Calories	Total fat (gm)	Saturated fat (gm)	Trans fats (gm)	Cholesterol (mg)	Sodium (mg)	Carbs (gm)
Hot & Sour Soup	1 cup	56	4	1	NA	NA	NA	86
Wonton Soup	1 cup	350	10	2	NA	NA	NA	44
Pin Rice Noodle Soup	1 Bowl	740	30	6	NA	NA	NA	91

P.F. Chang's® Continued

	Serving	Calories	Total fat (gm)	Saturated fat (gm)	Trans fats (gm)	Cholesterol (mg)	Sodium (mg)	Carbs (gm)
Salads w/ dressing								
Oriental Chicken Salad	1 salad	940	56	6	NA	NA	NA	42
Peanut Chicken Salad	1 salad	1080	69	9	NA	NA	NA	NA
Warm Duck Spinach Salad	1 salad	940	66	15	NA	NA	NA	NA
Nico's Favorite	1 salad	1230	96	26	NA	NA	NA	59
Sriracha Shrimp Salad	1 salad	1130	16	7	NA	NA	NA	163
Wild Alaskan Sockeye Salmon Salad	1 salad	610	35	5	NA	NA	NA	34
Traditional Entrées								
Almond Cashew Chicken	1 order	740	23	3.5	NA	NA	NA	61
Beef w/ broccoli	1 order	1120	65	16	NA	NA	NA	38
Crispy Honey Chicken	1 order	1110	39	4.5	NA	NA	NA	121
Lo Mein Beef	1 order	1790	80	22	NA	NA	NA	94
Lo Mein Chicken	1 order	1610	66	16	NA	NA	NA	97
Lo Mein Combo	1 order	1820	83	20	NA	NA	NA	98
Lo Mein Pork	1 order	1820	84	23	NA	NA	NA	95
Lo Mein Shrimp	1 order	1550	63	15	NA	NA	NA	97
Lo Mein Vegetable	1 order	1340	51	13	NA	NA	NA	96
Moo Goo Gai Pan	1 order	660	34	3.5	NA	NA	NA	32
Shrimp w/ lobster sauce	1 order	480	22	3.5	NA	NA	NA	24
Vegetarian Entrées								
Buddha's Feast (steamed)	1 order	200	1.5	1	NA	NA	NA	43
Buddha's Feast (stir-fried)	1 order	430	6	0	NA	NA	NA	80
Coconut-Curry Vegetables	1 order	690	46	24	NA	NA	NA	48
Garlic Snap Peas	1 order	210	10	1	NA	NA	NA	23
Ma Po Tofu	1 order	540	19	1	NA	NA	NA	51
Shanghai Cucumbers	1 order	120	6	1	NA	NA	NA	8
Sichuan-Style Asparagus	1 order	200	6	1	NA	NA	NA	34
Spicy Green Beans	1 order	610	40	6	NA	NA	NA	48
Spinach Stir-Fried w/ Garlic	1 order	140	6	1	NA	NA	NA	16
Stir-Fried Spicy Eggplant	1 order	600	34	4.5	NA	NA	NA	64
Chicken & Duck Entrées								
Cantonese Roasted Duck	1 order	900	54	18	NA	NA	NA	63
Chang's Spicy Chicken	1 order	930	37	5	NA	NA	NA	88
Chicken w/ Black Bean Sauce	1 order	700	25	4	NA	NA	NA	33
Ginger Chicken & Broccoli	1 order	660	26	4	NA	NA	NA	45
Kung Pao Chicken	1 order	1230	78	9	NA	NA	NA	58
Mango Chicken	1 order	730	19	2	NA	NA	NA	NA
Mu Shu Chicken	1 order	720	38	7	NA	NA	NA	50
Orange Peel Chicken	1 order	1280	60	7	NA	NA	NA	127
Philip's Better Lemon Chicken	1 order	1060	42	6	NA	NA	NA	113

Chicken & Duck Entrées continued

	Serving	Calories	Total fat (gm)	Saturated fat (gm)	Trans fats (gm)	Cholesterol (mg)	Sodium (mg)	Carbs (gm)
Spicy Ground Chicken & Eggplant	1 order	810	40	7	NA	NA	NA	73
Sweet & Sour Chicken	1 order	770	20	3.5	NA	NA	NA	107

Seafood Entrées

	Serving	Calories	Total fat (gm)	Saturated fat (gm)	Trans fats (gm)	Cholesterol (mg)	Sodium (mg)	Carbs (gm)
Wild Alaskan Sockeye Salmon w/ lemon pepper	1 order	670	36	5	NA	NA	NA	36
Wild Alaskan Sockeye Salmon Steamed w/ Ginger	1 order	790	50	8	NA	NA	NA	59
Cantonese Scallops	1 order	400	16	2	NA	NA	NA	26
Cantonese Shrimp	1 order	330	12	1	NA	NA	NA	21
Crispy Honey Shrimp	1 order	1380	64	8	NA	NA	NA	147
Hot Fish	1 order	1340	71	13	NA	NA	NA	111
Kung Pao Scallops	1 order	1130	56	6	NA	NA	NA	66
Kung Pao Shrimp	1 order	980	58	7	NA	NA	NA	58
Lemon Pepper Shrimp	1 order	710	36	4	NA	NA	NA	59
Lemon Scallops	1 order	950	27	2.5	NA	NA	NA	100
Oolong Marinated Sea Bass	1 order	520	12	2.5	NA	NA	NA	40
Orange Peel Shrimp	1 order	1020	41	4.5	NA	NA	NA	118
Shrimp w/ Candied Walnuts	1 order	1225	79	11	NA	NA	NA	74
Sichuan From the Sea Calamari	1 order	1000	39	7	NA	NA	NA	110
Sichuan From the Sea Scallops	1 order	1030	35	4	NA	NA	NA	98
Sichuan From the Sea Shrimp	1 order	730	37	4	NA	NA	NA	55
Spicy Salt & Pepper Prawns	1 order	850	50	6	NA	NA	NA	53

Beef & Pork Entrées

	Serving	Calories	Total fat (gm)	Saturated fat (gm)	Trans fats (gm)	Cholesterol (mg)	Sodium (mg)	Carbs (gm)
Beef a la Sichuan	1 order	1180	64	16	NA	NA	NA	56
Chendu Spiced Lamb	1 order	1060	75	16	NA	NA	NA	34
Mongolian Beef	1 order	1060	75	16	NA	NA	NA	34
Orange Peel Beef	1 order	1580	85	19	NA	NA	NA	115
Mu Shu Pork	1 order	880	51	12	NA	NA	NA	51
Sichuan-Style Pork	1 order	910	47	10	NA	NA	NA	NA
Sweet & Sour Pork	1 order	1100	46	14	NA	NA	NA	106
Wok Seared Lamb	1 order	1080	80	27	NA	NA	NA	29

Noodles, Meins & Rice Entrées

	Serving	Calories	Total fat (gm)	Saturated fat (gm)	Trans fats (gm)	Cholesterol (mg)	Sodium (mg)	Carbs (gm)
Cantonese Chow Fun Beef	1 order	1210	39	10	NA	NA	NA	142
Cantonese Chow Fun Chicken	1 order	1050	23	2.5	NA	NA	NA	146
Chow Mein Beef	1 order	790	26	7	NA	NA	NA	84
Chow Mein Pork	1 order	900	34	10	NA	NA	NA	83
Chow Mein Vegetable	1 order	470	4.5	1	NA	NA	NA	87
Dan-Dan Noodles	1 order	1090	30	5	NA	NA	NA	145
Double Pan-Fried Noodles-Beef	1 order	910	97	5	NA	NA	NA	116

	Serving	Calories	Total fat (gm)	Saturated fat (gm)	Trans fats (gm)	Cholesterol (mg)	Sodium (mg)	Carbs (gm)
Noodles, Meins & Rice Entrées continued								
Double Pan-Fried Noodles-Chicken	1 order	1080	47	7	NA	NA	NA	115
Double Pan-Fried Noodles-Vegetable	1 order	910	37	5	NA	NA	NA	116
Garlic Noodles	1 order	610	11	1.5	NA	NA	NA	111
Singapore Street Noodles	1 order	570	16	2	NA	NA	NA	91
Tams Noodles w/ Savory Beef & Shrimp	1 order	1700	94	15	NA	NA	NA	144
P. F. Chang's Fried Rice Chicken	1 order	1220	44	8	NA	NA	NA	151
P. F. Chang's Fried Rice Pork	1 order	1370	57	13	NA	NA	NA	150
P. F. Chang's Fried Rice Vegetable	1 order	1080	37	6	NA	NA	NA	154
Sichuan Chicken Chow Fun	1 order	690	19	2	NA	NA	NA	NA
Vegetable Chow Fun	1 order	880	8	0	NA	NA	NA	182
Cooked Brown Rice	1 order	350	3	1	NA	NA	NA	73
Cooked White Rice	1 order	410	1	0	NA	NA	NA	88
Desserts								
Banana Spring Rolls	1 order	950	52	18	NA	NA	NA	130
Flourless Chocolate Dome	1 order	570	26	8	NA	NA	NA	84
Great Wall of Chocolate	1 order	2240	89	21	NA	NA	NA	376
New York Style Cheesecake	1 order	950	55	34	NA	NA	NA	88
The Lucky 8	1 order	940	48	26	NA	NA	NA	105

Fast Food Factoid:

Rome wasn't built in a single day and a lifetime of eating habits can't be altered overnight. Choose just one GREEN food...you have to start sometime.

NOTES:

_____

_____

_____

_____

_____

_____

_____

Pizza Hut®

	Serving	Calories	Total fat (gm)	Saturated fat (gm)	Trans fats (gm)	Cholesterol (mg)	Sodium (mg)	Carbs (gm)
12" Lower Fat Pizza - 1 of 8 Slices								
Diced Chicken, Red Onion & Green Pepper	1 slice	170	5	2	0	15	460	NA
Diced Chicken, Mushroom & Jalapeño	1 slice	170	5	2	0	15	690	NA
Ham, Red Onion & Mushroom	1 slice	160	5	2	0	15	470	NA
Ham, Pineapple & Diced Tomato	1 slice	160	4	2	0	15	470	NA
Green Pepper, Red Onion & Diced Tomato	1 slice	150	4	2	0	10	360	NA
Tomato, Mushroom & Jalapeño	1 slice	150	4	2	0	10	590	NA
12" Hand-Tossed Pizza (medium) - 1 of 8 Slices								
Cheese	1 slice	240	8	5	0	25	520	25
Quartered Ham	1 slice	220	6	3	0	20	550	26
Pepperoni	1 slice	250	9	5	0	25	570	24
Supreme	1 slice	270	11	5	0	25	660	26
Chicken Supreme	1 slice	230	6	3	0	25	550	NA
Super Supreme	1 slice	300	13	6	0	35	780	NA
Meat Lover's	1 slice	300	13	6	0	35	760	25
Pepperoni Lover's	1 slice	300	13	7	0	40	710	NA
Sausage Lover's	1 slice	280	12	5	0	30	650	NA
Veggie Lover's	1 slice	220	6	3	0	15	490	26
12" Thin 'n Crispy Pizza (medium) - 1 of 8 Slices								
Cheese	1 slice	200	8	5	0	25	490	21
Italian Sausage	1 slice	230	11	5	0	30	620	23
Meat Lovers	1 slice	310	18	7	1	45	1010	22
Quartered Ham	1 slice	180	6	3	0	20	530	23
Pepperoni	1 slice	210	10	5	0	25	550	21
Supreme	1 slice	240	11	5	1	25	640	22
Chicken Supreme	1 slice	200	7	4	0	25	520	NA
Super Supreme	1 slice	260	13	6	1	35	760	NA
Veggie Lovers	1 slice	180	7	3	0	15	550	23
12" Pan Pizza (medium) - 1 of 8 Slices								
Cheese	1 slice	280	13	5	0	25	500	27
Italian Sausage	1 slice	300	15	5	0	30	610	28
Meat Lovers	1 slice	370	22	8	0	45	990	28
Quartered Ham	1 slice	260	11	4	0	20	540	28
Pepperoni	1 slice	290	15	5	0	25	560	29
Supreme	1 slice	320	16	6	0	25	650	28
Chicken Supreme	1 slice	280	12	4	0	25	530	28
Super Supreme	1 slice	340	18	6	0	35	760	NA
Veggie Lovers	1 slice	250	11	4	0	15	530	28

Pizza Hut®
Continued

	Serving	Calories	Total fat (gm)	Saturated fat (gm)	Trans fats (gm)	Cholesterol (mg)	Sodium (mg)	Carbs (gm)
14" Stuffed Crust Pizza (large) - 1 of 8 Slices								
Cheese	1 slice	360	13	8	1	40	920	37
Italian Sausage	1 slice	410	20	9	2	50	1160	38
Meat Lovers	1 slice	520	29	12	2	75	1690	37
Quartered Ham	1 slice	340	11	6	0	40	960	38
Pepperoni	1 slice	370	15	8	1	45	970	35
Supreme	1 slice	400	16	8	1	45	1070	37
Chicken Supreme	1 slice	380	13	7	1	40	1020	NA
Super Supreme	1 slice	440	20	9	1	50	1270	NA
Veggie Lovers	1 slice	340	14	7	2	35	1030	37
16" Full House Pizza (large) - 1 of 8 Slices								
Cheese	1 slice	280	12	6	0	25	760	30
Italian Sausage	1 slice	300	14	5	0	30	720	32
Meat Lovers	1 slice	370	20	8	0	45	1090	31
Quartered Ham	1 slice	260	10	4	0	25	790	32
Pepperoni	1 slice	290	13	5	0	25	810	30
Supreme	1 slice	310	15	6	0	30	890	31
Chicken Supreme	1 slice	270	10	4	0	25	770	NA
Super Supreme	1 slice	330	16	6	0	35	1000	NA
Veggie Lovers	1 slice	260	10	4	0	20	650	31
6" Personal Pan Pizza - 1 of 4 Slices								
Cheese	1 slice	160	7	3	1	15	310	69
Italian Sausage	Whole	690	33	12	1	70	1530	71
Meat Lovers	Whole	890	49	18	1	115	2460	70
Quartered Ham	1 slice	150	6	2	1	15	330	70
Pepperoni	1 slice	170	8	3	1	15	340	67
Supreme	1 slice	190	9	4	1	20	420	70
Chicken Supreme	1 slice	160	6	3	1	15	320	NA
Super Supreme	1 slice	200	10	4	1	20	480	NA
Veggie Lovers	Whole	560	22	8	0	40	1250	70
6" Carb Tracker Pizza - 1 of 8 Slices								
Pepperoni	1 pizza	520	29	12	0	60	1550	NA
Pepperoni & Mushroom	1 pizza	490	25	11	0	55	1400	NA
Meat Lover's	1 pizza	740	46	19	0	110	2170	NA
Appetizers, Dipping Sauces & Cinnamon Sticks								
Breadsticks	1 item	150	6	1	0	0	220	20
Cheese Breadsticks	1 item	200	10	4	0	15	340	21
Hot Wings	2 items	110	6	2	0	70	450	1
Mild Wings	2 items	110	7	2	0	70	320	2
Breadstick Dipping Sauce	3 oz.	50	0	0	0	0	370	8

Pizza Hut®
Continued

Appetizers, Dipping Sauces & Cinnamon Sticks continued

	Serving	Calories	Total fat (gm)	Saturated fat (gm)	Trans fats (gm)	Cholesterol (mg)	Sodium (mg)	Carbs (gm)
Wing Blue Cheese Dipping Sauce	1.5 oz.	230	24	5	0	25	550	3
Wing Ranch Dipping Sauce	1.5 oz.	210	22	4	0	10	340	3
Cinnamon Sticks	2 items	170	5	1	0	0	170	27
White Icing Dipping Cup	2 oz.	190	0	0	0	0	0	47
Apple Dessert Pizza	1 slice	260	5	1	1	0	290	52
Cherry Dessert Pizza	1 slice	260	5	1	1	0	280	47

Ponderosa Steakhouse®
Does not provide nutrition information.

Popeyes Chicken & Biscuits®

Mild Chicken

	Serving	Calories	Total fat	Saturated fat	Trans fats	Cholesterol	Sodium	Carbs
Wing	63g	150	10	3.5	0	90	510	5
Leg	75g	110	7	2.5	0	110	500	3
Thigh	123g	280	20	7	0.5	150	890	7
Breast	195g	350	20	7	0.5	195	1380	8
Strips (2 pcs.)	116g	250	10	4.5	0.5	55	1260	16

Mild Chicken (skinless, breading removed)

	Serving	Calories	Total fat	Saturated fat	Trans fats	Cholesterol	Sodium	Carbs
Wing	51g	40	1.5	0.5	0	70	470	0
Leg	61g	50	2	0.5	0	100	370	0
Thigh	92g	80	4	1	0	125	690	0
Breast	148g	120	2	1	0	145	960	0
Strips (2 pcs.)	94g	130	2.5	1	0	50	920	3

Spicy Chicken

	Serving	Calories	Total fat	Saturated fat	Trans fats	Cholesterol	Sodium	Carbs
Wing	63g	140	9	3.5	0	85	370	5
Leg	75g	100	5	2	0	85	420	3
Thigh	123g	300	24	8	0.5	145	690	7
Breast	195g	360	22	8	0.5	185	1090	8
Strips (2 pcs.)	116g	270	11	4.5	0.5	55	1370	21

Spicy Chicken (skinless, breading removed)

	Serving	Calories	Total fat	Saturated fat	Trans fats	Cholesterol	Sodium	Carbs
Cajun Wing Segments	6 Pieces	595	43	15	2	260	1274	0
Wing	51g	40	2	3.5	0	80	310	0
Leg	61g	50	1.5	2	0	70	260	2
Thigh	92g	80	3	8	0	125	450	1
Breast	148g	120	2	8	0	135	730	5
Strips (2 pcs.)	94g	150	4	4.5	0	55	880	19

Popeyes Chicken & Biscuits®
Continued

Naked Chicken Strips

	Serving	Calories	Total fat (gm)	Saturated fat (gm)	Trans fats (gm)	Cholesterol (mg)	Sodium (mg)	Carbs (gm)
Strips (3 pcs.)	118g	170	5	2	NA	80	790	NA

Items

	Serving	Calories	Total fat (gm)	Saturated fat (gm)	Trans fats (gm)	Cholesterol (mg)	Sodium (mg)	Carbs (gm)
Deluxe Tame w/ mayonnaise	265g	630	31	8	1	71	1500	53
Deluxe Tame w/o mayonnaise	237g	480	15	6	0.5	55	1340	54
Shrimp (fully dressed)	253g	740	40	10	NA	100	1860	NA
Catfish (fully dressed)	229g	640	35	9	NA	45	1330	NA

Seafood

	Serving	Calories	Total fat (gm)	Saturated fat (gm)	Trans fats (gm)	Cholesterol (mg)	Sodium (mg)	Carbs (gm)
Popcorn Shrimp	85g	280	16	6	1	95	710	22
Fried Crawfish	106g	370	21	9	NA	185	830	NA
Fried Catfish	104g	300	18	7	NA	55	820	NA

Popeyes Louisiana Legends™

	Serving	Calories	Total fat (gm)	Saturated fat (gm)	Trans fats (gm)	Cholesterol (mg)	Sodium (mg)	Carbs (gm)
Chicken Sausage Jambalaya	151g	660	33	9	3	32	370	60
Smothered Chicken	151g	630	24	6	0	23	743	72
Chicken Étouffée	151g	480	30	9	0	20	420	18
Crawfish Étouffée	151g	540	15	3	0	48	530	75

Sides

	Serving	Calories	Total fat (gm)	Saturated fat (gm)	Trans fats (gm)	Cholesterol (mg)	Sodium (mg)	Carbs (gm)
Buttermilk Biscuits	60g	240	13	7	0	0	500	26
French Fries	88g	310	17	7	1	7	632	35
Corn on the Cob	220g	190	2	0.5	0	0	25	37
Mashed Potatoes, w/o gravy	113g	100	3	1	0.5	0	380	17
Mashed Potatoes & Gravy	142g	130	4	2	0.5	5	570	18
Red Beans & Rice	174g	320	19	6	0	20	700	31
Cajun Rice	117g	170	6	2	0	60	440	22
Coleslaw	138g	260	23	3.5	0	15	260	14
Green Beans	100g	70	1	0	0	5	480	14
Collard Greens	116g	50	2	1	NA	5	500	NA
Cinnamon Apple Turnover	86g	250	12	4	1.5	5	290	34

Quiznos Sub®
Does not provide nutrition information.

Red Lobster®
Does not provide nutrition information.

Red Robin Burgers & Spirits Emporium®
Does not provide nutrition information.

Romano's Macaroni Grill®

	Serving	Calories	Total fat (gm)	Saturated fat (gm)	Trans fats (gm)	Cholesterol (mg)	Sodium (mg)	Carbs (gm)
Antipasti								
Calamari Fritti	1 item	1210	78	13	NA	NA	4170	66
Mozzarella Alla Caprese (half order)	3 items	260	21	7	NA	NA	360	NA
Mozzarella Alla Caprese (full order)	5 items	460	38	12	NA	NA	660	NA
Mozzarella Fritta	1 item	880	63	18	NA	NA	1810	54
Mushroom Ravioli	1 item	820	60	24	NA	NA	1130	NA
Mussels Tarantina	1 item	980	68	11	NA	NA	1280	NA
Peasant Bread	1 loaf	500	12	1	NA	NA	2020	89
Prosciutto Bruschetta	1 item	760	42	22	NA	NA	1240	NA
Romano's Sampler (Tomato Bruschetta, Mozzarella Fritta & Calamari)	1 item	1260	86	25	NA	NA	2840	31
Fried Calamari	1 item	350	23	4	NA	NA	600	59
Fried Mozzarella	1 item	480	32	10	NA	NA	70	32
Romano's Sampler - Garnish only	1 item	60	4	1	NA	NA	400	4
Shrimp & Artichoke Dip	1 item	1030	52	24	NA	NA	3600	88
Crab Stuffed Mushrooms	1 item	740	36	9	NA	NA	1110	71
Tomato Bruschetta	1 item	820	54	6	NA	NA	1790	75
Wood-Fired Pizzas & Calzonettos								
BBQ Chicken Pizza	1 pizza	950	27	14	NA	NA	2790	135
Pizza Margherita	1 pizza	950	36	18	NA	NA	2160	123
Grilled Chicken Caesar Calzonetto	1 order	1500	90	22	NA	NA	3500	124
½ Grilled Chicken Caesar Calzonetto	½ order	750	45	11	NA	NA	1750	62
Grilled Chicken Calzonetto	1 Sandwich	1540	88	23	NA	NA	2740	NA
Sandwiches								
Brick-Oven Meatball Sandwich	1 Sandwich	1890	115	38	NA	NA	460	149
Roasted Chicken & Cheese	1 Sandwich	1630	91	23	NA	NA	2520	128
Insalata (salads)								
Caesar della Casa	1 order	260	21	5	NA	NA	650	13
Garden della Casa w/o dressing	1 order	130	5	2	NA	NA	460	15
Garden della Casa	1 order	240	15	4	NA	NA	900	20
Chicken Caesar	1 order	840	64	15	NA	NA	1660	24
Chicken Florentine	1 order	840	53	9	NA	NA	5450	62
Chicken Florentine w/o dressing	1 order	490	19	4	NA	NA	4930	20
Insalata Bleu Salad	1 order	650	55	14	NA	NA	1460	13
Insalata Bleu Salad w/o dressing	1 order	440	36	12	NA	NA	970	9
Insalata Bleu Salad w/ chicken	1 order	770	57	15	NA	NA	1520	13
Insalata Bleu Salad w/ chicken, w/o dressing	1 order	570	38	12	NA	NA	1020	9

Romano's Macaroni Grill®
Continued

Insalata (salads) continued

	Serving	Calories	Total fat (gm)	Saturated fat (gm)	Trans fats (gm)	Cholesterol (mg)	Sodium (mg)	Carbs (gm)
½ Insalata Bleu Salad w/ entrée, dressing	1 order	380	32	8	NA	NA	860	NA
Insalata Rossa Salad	1 order	440	6	2	NA	NA	1430	NA
Insalata Rossa Salad w/o dressing	1 order	340	6	2	NA	NA	1430	NA
Mozarella Alla Caprese	1/2 order	260	21	7	NA	NA	40	9
Parmesan Crusted Chicken	1 order	1190	63	17	NA	NA	3230	60
Parmesan Crusted Chicken w/out Dressing	1 order	1060	49	15	NA	NA	2880	59
Seared Sea Scallops	1 order	1320	91	25	NA	NA	2860	23
Seared Sea Scallops w/out Dressing	1 order	1050	68	22	NA	NA	2810	22
Steak & Arugula	1 order	890	71	18	NA	NA	3290	11
Steak & Arugula w/out Dressing	1 order	570	37	13	NA	NA	2530	9

Soups

	Serving	Calories	Total fat (gm)	Saturated fat (gm)	Trans fats (gm)	Cholesterol (mg)	Sodium (mg)	Carbs (gm)
Lentil Bean	1 bowl	360	9	2	NA	NA	1580	NA
Lentil Bean	1 cup	180	5	1	NA	NA	800	NA
Minestrone	1 bowl	510	23	4	NA	NA	2130	NA
Minestrone	1 cup	380	20	4	NA	NA	1130	NA
Pasta Fagioli	1 bowl	760	31	5	NA	NA	1960	NA
Pasta Fagioli	1 cup	450	23	4	NA	NA	1010	NA
Chicken Toscana Soup	1 bowl	510	32	15	NA	NA	3240	36
Chicken Toscana Soup	1 cup	260	16	8	NA	NA	1640	18
Tomato Tortellini Soup	1 cup	250	11	5	NA	NA	1170	NA

Sides

	Serving	Calories	Total fat (gm)	Saturated fat (gm)	Trans fats (gm)	Cholesterol (mg)	Sodium (mg)	Carbs (gm)
Pasta Salad	1 Side	310	16	3	NA	NA	520	69
Garlic Mashed Potatoes	1 Side	280	14	3	NA	NA	640	35
Grilled Asparagus	1 Side	30	1	0	NA	NA	590	4
Romanos Parmesan Chips	1 Side	660	51	11	NA	NA	390	39
Sauteéd Broccoli	1 Side	260	22	4	NA	NA	350	12

From the Grill (includes sides)

	Serving	Calories	Total fat (gm)	Saturated fat (gm)	Trans fats (gm)	Cholesterol (mg)	Sodium (mg)	Carbs (gm)
Boursin Filet	1 order	1120	83	37	NA	NA	2440	39
Honey Balsamic Chicken	1 order	1560	68	12	NA	NA	3000	94
Grilled Pork Chops	1 order	1800	107	43	NA	NA	4950	93
Tuscan Ribeye	1 order	1070	76	31	NA	NA	4720	40
Chicken & Shrimp Scalloppine, Lunch	1 order	1260	89	34	NA	NA	3150	66
Chicken Portobello	1 order	1020	65	11	NA	NA	6980	61
Chicken Sorrentino	1 order	1050	46	10	NA	NA	1660	85
Grilled Salmon	1 order	1360	84	10	NA	NA	7100	79
Grilled Halibut	1 order	840	44	12	NA	NA	1430	56

	Serving	Calories	Total fat (gm)	Saturated fat (gm)	Trans fats (gm)	Cholesterol (mg)	Sodium (mg)	Carbs (gm)
From the Grill (includes sides) continued								
Tuscan Ribeye	1 order	1000	66	23	NA	NA	5180	40
Pellame (chicken)								
Chicken Scaloppine (lunch)	1 order	1010	64	28	NA	NA	2650	65
Chicken Scaloppine (dinner)	1 order	1110	71	30	NA	NA	2870	68
Chicken Parmigiano (lunch)	1 order	910	37	19	NA	NA	2030	89
Chicken Parmigiano (dinner)	1 order	1490	68	35	NA	NA	3510	126
Chicken Marsala (lunch)	1 order	1015	62	22	NA	NA	2060	73
Chicken Marsala (dinner)	1 order	1130	70	24	NA	NA	2300	76
Pesce (seafood)								
Shrimp Diavolo	1 order	1150	74	10	NA	NA	2480	NA
Angelini di Mare	1 order	1380	87	40	NA	NA	1540	NA
Shrimp Portofino (lunch)	1 order	1090	79	29	NA	NA	1830	65
Shrimp Portofino (dinner)	1 order	1130	80	29	NA	NA	1880	66
Carni (beef)								
Veal Saltimbocca	1 order	1220	70	41	NA	NA	2760	NA
Veal Marsala	1 order	1090	47	20	NA	NA	2680	132
Veal Parmesan	1 order	1260	63	11	NA	NA	2640	116
Pasta								
Capellini Pomodoro (lunch)	1 order	750	37	6	NA	NA	920	NA
Capellini Pomodoro (dinner)	1 order	880	38	6	NA	NA	1150	NA
Capellini Pomodoro w/ chicken (lunch)	1 order	870	39	7	NA	NA	980	NA
Capellini Pomodoro w/ chicken (dinner)	1 order	1000	41	7	NA	NA	1210	NA
Capellini Pomodoro w/ shrimp (lunch	1 order	830	37	6	NA	NA	1020	NA
Capellini Pomodoro w/ shrimp (dinner)	1 order	950	39	6	NA	NA	1250	NA
Carmela's Chicken Rigatoni (lunch)	1 order	1030	65	27	NA	NA	1290	64
Carmela's Chicken Rigatoni (dinner)	1 order	1320	87	34	NA	NA	1550	84
Eggplant Parmesan (lunch)	1 order	1070	56	33	NA	NA	2150	102
Eggplant Parmesan (dinner)	1 order	1230	64	35	NA	NA	2540	118
Fettuccine Alfredo (dinner)	1 order	1130	82	53	NA	NA	1200	68
Fettuccine Alfredo w/ shrimp (lunch & dinner)	1 order	1330	96	56	NA	NA	1340	70
Fettuccine Alfredo w/ chicken (lunch & dinner)	1 order	1370	98	56	NA	NA	1300	68
Lasagna Bolognese (lunch)	1 order	940	52	28	NA	NA	2130	NA
Mama's Trio	1 order	1490	73	40	NA	NA	3540	81
Penne Arrabbiata (lunch)	1 order	1000	73	32	NA	NA	2450	NA

Romano's Macaroni Grill®
Continued

Pasta continued

	Serving	Calories	Total fat (gm)	Saturated fat (gm)	Trans fats (gm)	Cholesterol (mg)	Sodium (mg)	Carbs (gm)
Penne Arrabbiata (dinner)	1 order	1090	73	32	NA	NA	2900	NA
Penne Arrabbiata w/ chicken (lunch)	1 order	1120	75	32	NA	NA	2510	NA
Penne Arrabbiata w/ chicken (dinner)	1 order	1220	76	33	NA	NA	2960	NA
Penne Arrabbiata w/ shrimp (lunch)	1 order	1080	73	32	NA	NA	2550	NA
Penne Arrabbiata w/ shrimp (dinner)	1 order	1170	74	32	NA	NA	3000	NA
Pasta Milano (lunch)	1 order	890	47	16	NA	NA	1460	83
Pasta Milano (dinner)	1 order	1080	55	20	NA	NA	1910	108
Penne Rustica (lunch)	1 order	1260	70	31	NA	NA	2400	76
Penne Rustica (dinner)	1 order	1480	78	36	NA	NA	2830	101
Sausage & Pepper Classico (lunch)	1 order	770	45	24	NA	NA	2020	NA
Sausage & Pepper Classico (dinner)	1 order	860	45	24	NA	NA	2470	NA
Spaghetti & Meatballs w/ tomato sauce (lunch)	1 order	1080	63	34	NA	NA	3350	NA
Spaghetti & Meatballs w/ tomato sauce (dinner)	1 order	1430	81	41	NA	NA	4530	NA
Spaghetti & Meatballs w/ meat sauce (lunch)	1 order	1290	79	39	NA	NA	3590	NA
Spaghetti & Meatballs w/ meat sauce (dinner)	1 order	2270	115	56	NA	NA	5330	NA

Stuffed Pasta

	Serving	Calories	Total fat (gm)	Saturated fat (gm)	Trans fats (gm)	Cholesterol (mg)	Sodium (mg)	Carbs (gm)
Lobster Ravioli	1 order	1090	79	54	NA	NA	1910	55
Chicken Cannelloni (lunch)	1 order	690	37	22	NA	NA	1910	42
Chicken Cannelloni (dinner)	1 order	1030	55	34	NA	NA	2830	62
Twice Baked Lasagna w/ meatballs	1 order	1420	85	41	NA	NA	3920	81

Sensible Fare

	Serving	Calories	Total fat (gm)	Saturated fat (gm)	Trans fats (gm)	Cholesterol (mg)	Sodium (mg)	Carbs (gm)
Simple Salmon	1 order	630	42	7	NA	NA	880	5
Chicken Toscana	1 order	550	27	6	NA	NA	2390	NA
Mediterranean Shrimp	1 order	240	2	0	NA	NA	2470	NA
Pollo Magro "Skinny Chicken"	1 order	310	5	1	NA	NA	770	29
Steak & Arugula Salad	1 order	990	80	23	NA	NA	2010	11
Steak & Arugula Salad w/o dressing	1 order	670	46	17	NA	NA	1260	9

Kid's

	Serving	Calories	Total fat (gm)	Saturated fat (gm)	Trans fats (gm)	Cholesterol (mg)	Sodium (mg)	Carbs (gm)
Crunchin' Corn Dog	1 item	250	17	4	NA	NA	260	NA
Cheeseoli	1 order	340	14	7	NA	NA	560	NA
Chicken Fingerias only	1 order	790	61	10	NA	NA	1790	NA
Fettuccine Alfredo	1 order	530	26	14	NA	NA	1240	53

Romano's Macaroni Grill®
Continued

Kid's continued	Serving	Calories	Total fat (gm)	Saturated fat (gm)	Trans fats (gm)	Cholesterol (mg)	Sodium (mg)	Carbs (gm)
Grilled Cheese only	1 order	590	47	17	NA	NA	1310	NA
Grilled Chicken & Broccoli	1 order	380	5	2	NA	NA	1920	51
Lasagna	1 order	480	26	14	NA	NA	1130	NA
Macaroni 'n Cheese	1 order	580	31	20	NA	NA	1870	30
Mona Lisa's Cheese Masterpizza	1 order	770	23	12	NA	NA	1820	120
Mona Lisa's Pepperoni Masterpizza	1 order	850	30	15	NA	NA	2080	120
Spaghettini w/ meat sauce	1 order	320	7	3	NA	NA	670	NA
Spaghetti & Meatballs w/ tomato sauce	1 order	500	20	8	NA	NA	1520	58
Spaghetti & Meatballs w/ meat sauce	1 order	550	24	10	NA	NA	1550	56
Kid's Sides								
Broccoli Crowns	4 oz.	40	1	0	NA	NA	110	11
Macaroni 'n Cheese (side only)	3 oz.	350	18	12	NA	NA	1120	30
Shoestring Fries	4 oz.	250	15	3	NA	NA	390	27
Caesar della Casa	1 order	170	12	3	NA	NA	460	11
Garden della Casa w/ dressing	1 order	150	9	2	NA	NA	590	9
Desserts								
Café Latte Cheesecake	1 order	1500	96	56	NA	NA	710	NA
Dessert, Dessert, Dessert	1 order	1940	102	53	NA	NA	1120	NA
Dessert Ravioli	1 order	1720	89	43	NA	NA	770	223
Lemon Passion	1 order	1270	69	38	NA	NA	790	149
New York Cheesecake	1 order	1080	76	46	NA	NA	630	75
New York Cheesecake w/ caramel fudge sauce	1 order	1760	113	66	NA	NA	710	169
New York Cheesecake w/ strawberry sauce	1 order	1150	76	46	NA	NA	630	NA
Smothered Chocolate Cake	1 order	1450	90	44	NA	NA	930	140
Strawberries Zabaglione	1 order	450	34	21	NA	NA	40	NA
Tiramisu	1 order	1440	65	34	NA	NA	550	89
Fresh Strawberries (Kid's)	1 order	40	0	0	NA	NA	10	NA
Ice Cream Scoop (Kid's)	1 order	400	23	14	NA	NA	100	43

Ruby Tuesday®
Ruby Tuesday does have some nutrition information, but not enough to make a valid guideline. Consequently, all Ruby Tuesday foods were left out of this guide.

Sbarro®

	Serving	Calories	Total fat (gm)	Saturated fat (gm)	Trans fats (gm)	Cholesterol (mg)	Sodium (mg)	Carbs (gm)
Gourmet Pizza (medium) - 1 of 8 Slices								
Cheese	1 slice	660	21	NA	NA	40	1460	NA
Mushroom	1 slice	610	20	NA	NA	20	1600	NA
Meat Delight	1 slice	780	29	NA	NA	80	2250	NA
Broccoli & Spinach	1 slice	720	28	NA	NA	30	1540	NA
Ham, Pineapple & Bacon	1 slice	680	21	NA	NA	45	1820	NA
Mushroom & Spinach	1 slice	710	27	NA	NA	30	1680	NA
Tomato & Basil	1 slice	700	25	NA	NA	40	1650	NA
Low-Carb Pizza (medium) - 1 of 8 Slices								
Cheese	1 slice	410	14	NA	NA	25	640	NA
Pepperoni	1 slice	420	14	NA	NA	60	940	NA
Sausage	1 slice	560	35	NA	NA	95	1300	NA
Traditional Pizza (medium) - 1 of 8 Slices								
Cheese	1 slice	460	13	NA	NA	30	1080	NA
Pepperoni	1 slice	730	37	NA	NA	75	2200	NA
Sausage	1 slice	670	31	NA	NA	80	1810	NA
Supreme	1 slice	630	27	NA	NA	60	1720	NA
White	1 slice	570	23	NA	NA	55	1150	NA
Chicken Vegetable	1 slice	530	17	NA	NA	45	1260	NA
Mushroom	1 slice	460	14	NA	NA	20	1310	NA
Fresh Tomato	1 slice	450	14	NA	NA	25	1040	NA
Stuffed Pizza (medium) - 1 of 8 Slices								
Stuffed Spinach & Broccoli	1 slice	790	34	NA	NA	50	1610	NA
Stuffed Pepperoni	1 slice	960	42	NA	NA	115	3200	NA
Stuffed Philly Cheesesteak	1 slice	830	33	NA	NA	70	2090	NA
Salads								
Garden Salad	1 salad	35	0	NA	NA	0	15	NA
Fruit Salad	1 salad	130	1	NA	NA	0	15	NA
Caesar Salad	1 salad	80	5	NA	NA	5	200	NA
Cucumber & Tomato Salad	1 salad	130	11	NA	NA	0	85	NA
Stringbean & Tomato Salad	1 salad	100	7	NA	NA	0	80	NA
Pasta Primavera	1 salad	190	10	NA	NA	0	1180	NA
Greek Salad	1 salad	60	5	NA	NA	10	130	NA
Items								
Spinach, Tomato, Broccoli Stromboli	1 item	680	24	NA	NA	35	1420	NA
Pepperoni Stromboli	1 item	890	44	NA	NA	80	2470	NA
Cheese Calzone	1 item	770	28	NA	NA	90	1410	NA
Dinners (entrée only unless otherwise noted)								
Baked Ziti w/ sauce	14 oz.	700	41	NA	NA	135	1220	NA

Sbarro® Continued

Dinners continued

	Serving	Calories	Total fat (gm)	Saturated fat (gm)	Trans fats (gm)	Cholesterol (mg)	Sodium (mg)	Carbs (gm)
Meat Lasagna	13 oz.	650	37	NA	NA	130	1130	NA
Chicken Parmesan	11 oz.	520	22	NA	NA	175	750	NA
Chicken Francese	11 oz.	640	38	NA	NA	175	590	NA
Chicken Vesuvio	11 oz.	690	43	NA	NA	225	810	NA
Chicken Portofino	11.75 oz.	730	48	NA	NA	225	790	NA
Eggplant Rollatini w/ cheese	10.5 oz.	580	38	NA	NA	50	900	NA
Spaghetti w/ sauce	20 oz.	820	28	NA	NA	0	890	NA
Spaghetti w/ meatballs	18 oz.	680	25	NA	NA	15	1720	NA
Spaghetti w/ chicken parmesan	15 oz.	930	36	NA	NA	175	950	NA
Spaghetti w/ chicken francese	15 oz.	800	37	NA	NA	110	860	NA
Spaghetti w/ chicken vesuvio	15 oz.	850	41	NA	NA	145	1100	NA
Meatballs	3.25 oz.	140	9	NA	NA	30	880	NA
Sausage & Peppers	10 oz.	410	30	NA	NA	55	1340	NA
Penne w/ sausage & peppers	14 oz.	710	49	NA	NA	130	1690	NA
Pasta Milano	20 oz.	640	32	NA	NA	175	740	NA
Mixed Vegetables	7 oz.	190	15	NA	NA	0	330	NA

Schlotzsky's Deli®

Sandwiches

	Serving	Calories	Total fat (gm)	Saturated fat (gm)	Trans fats (gm)	Cholesterol (mg)	Sodium (mg)	Carbs (gm)
The Original	small	525	24	NA	1	85	1781	52
Ham & Cheese Original	small	512	19	NA	1	80	2323	54
Turkey Original	small	583	24	NA	1	101	2161	54
Smoked Turkey Breast	small	500	7	NA	0	59	1805	53
Angus Roast Beef & Cheese	medium	780	33	NA	1	119	2102	73
Turkey Bacon Club	medium	770	29	NA	1	122	2450	76
Grilled Chicken Breast	medium	545	7	NA	0	86	1702	80
Chicken Breast	medium	509	6	NA	0	67	1909	77
Fresh Veggie	medium	483	12	NA	0	23	1153	77

Reuben Items (small)

	Serving	Calories	Total fat (gm)	Saturated fat (gm)	Trans fats (gm)	Cholesterol (mg)	Sodium (mg)	Carbs (gm)
Corned Beef on Dark Rye	1 item	534	20	NA	0	95	2568	77
Angus Pastrami Reuben	1 item	629	27	NA	1	100	1591	58
Turkey on Dark Rye	1 item	554	23	NA	1	95	2684	54

Specialty Items (small)

	Serving	Calories	Total fat (gm)	Saturated fat (gm)	Trans fats (gm)	Cholesterol (mg)	Sodium (mg)	Carbs (gm)
BLT	1 item	379	15	NA	0	28	1010	50
Chicken Club	1 item	458	15	NA	NA	NA	1591	NA
Corned Beef on Dark Rye	1 item	393	8	NA	0	36	1924	77
Roast Beef	1 item	418	10	NA	NA	NA	1622	NA
Roast Beef & Cheese	1 item	586	23	NA	1	85	2040	50

Schlotzsky's Deli® Continued

	Serving	Calories	Total fat (gm)	Saturated fat (gm)	Trans fats (gm)	Cholesterol (mg)	Sodium (mg)	Carbs (gm)
Specialty Items (small) continued								
The Philly	1 item	571	21	NA	NA	NA	2064	NA
Albacore Tuna Melt on Wheat	1 item	529	21	NA	0	51	1677	76
Turkey & Bacon Club on Wheat	1 item	571	24	NA	1	91	2038	53
Turkey Guacamole	1 item	423	12	NA	0	36	1789	52
Vegetable Club	1 item	367	13	NA	NA	NA	1036	NA
Western Vegetarian	1 item	425	20	NA	NA	NA	816	NA
Chipotle Chicken	1 item	379	10	NA	0	55	1094	50
Grilled Chicken & Pesto	1 item	413	10	NA	0	61	988	52
Dijon Chicken	1 item	391	7	NA	0	46	1539	54
Angus Corned Beef	1 item	395	9	NA	0	36	1568	53
Light & Flavorful Items (small)								
Chicken Breast	1 item	337	3	NA	NA	NA	1588	NA
Dijon Chicken on Wheat	1 item	329	4	NA	NA	NA	1456	NA
Pesto Chicken	1 item	346	6	NA	NA	NA	1297	NA
Albacore Tuna on Wheat	1 item	334	7	NA	NA	NA	1230	NA
Smoked Turkey Breast	1 item	335	5	NA	NA	NA	1427	NA
The Vegetarian on Wheat	1 item	324	7	NA	NA	NA	996	NA
Bun Choices (small)								
Sourdough	1 bun	225	1	NA	NA	NA	582	NA
Dark Rye	1 bun	218	1	NA	NA	NA	546	NA
Jalapeño Cheese	1 bun	235	3	NA	NA	NA	630	NA
Wheat	1 bun	226	2	NA	NA	NA	583	NA
8" Sourdough Crust Pizza								
Original Combination	1 pizza	625	23	NA	NA	54	2068	76
Bacon, Tomato & Mushroom	1 pizza	611	22	NA	NA	NA	1966	NA
BBQ Chicken & Jalapeno	1 pizza	684	16	NA	0	81	2321	98
Chicken & Pesto	1 pizza	649	19	NA	NA	NA	2187	NA
Thai Chicken	1 pizza	663	17	NA	NA	NA	2297	NA
Double Cheese	1 pizza	580	19	NA	NA	NA	1791	NA
Double Cheese & Pepperoni	1 pizza	685	30	NA	1	71	1740	74
Mediterranean	1 pizza	560	20	NA	0	85	1580	74
Three Meat	1 pizza	805	39	NA	NA	NA	2797	NA
Fresh Tomato & Pesto	1 pizza	539	16	NA	NA	NA	1670	NA
Vegetarian Special	1 pizza	551	17	NA	NA	NA	1812	NA
Wraps								
Asian Almond Chicken	1 wrap	459	7	NA	NA	NA	2391	NA
Salsa Chicken w/ cheddar	1 wrap	460	17	NA	NA	NA	1419	NA
Zesty Albacore Tuna	1 wrap	311	7	NA	NA	NA	1226	NA

Schlotzsky's Deli® Continued

	Serving	Calories	Total fat (gm)	Saturated fat (gm)	Trans fats (gm)	Cholesterol (mg)	Sodium (mg)	Carbs (gm)
Kid's Meals (w/o cookie or drink)								
Cheese Pizza	1 pizza	479	13	NA	0	24	1059	73
Pepperoni Pizza	1 pizza	523	17	NA	0	33	1245	73
Cheese item	1 item	397	15	NA	1	40	1037	48
Ham & Cheese item	1 item	431	16	NA	1	50	1154	49
Turkey Sandwich	1 item	298	5	NA	0	23	837	49
Salads								
Gilled Chicken Caesar	1 salad	221	8	NA	0	65	759	12
Caesar	1 salad	103	5	NA	0	6	289	10
Garden	1 salad	51	1	NA	0	0	291	12
Turkey Chef	1 salad	239	15	NA	0	77	1299	15
Baby Spinach & Feta	1 salad	197	15	NA	0	27	447	10
Chicken Salad	1 salad	292	15	NA	0	93	898	12
Greek	1 salad	137	8	NA	0	29	655	13
Ham & Turkey Chef	1 salad	249	13	NA	0	63	1424	14

Shoney's®

	Serving	Calories	Total fat (gm)	Saturated fat (gm)	Trans fats (gm)	Cholesterol (mg)	Sodium (mg)	Carbs (gm)
Dinner Entrées								
Roast Beef Platter	1 order	880	30	12	NA	136	3253	NA
Grandma's Meatloaf w/ glaze	1 order	1092	47	15	NA	188	2276	NA
Grandma's Meatloaf w/ gravy	1 order	1089	49	16	NA	189	2451	NA
Original Country Fried Steak	1 order	1151	62	14	NA	107	4073	NA
Grilled Liver 'n Onions	1 order	711	22	4	NA	683	1115	NA
Ham Steak Dinner	1 order	667	26	6	NA	100	3210	NA
Baked Whitefish	1 order	507	8	1	NA	94	2231	NA
Cajun Whitefish	1 order	480	10	1	NA	73	883	NA
Dinner Sides								
Mashed Potatoes w/ gravy	1 order	223	10	2	NA	7	575	NA
Corn	1 order	173	9	1	NA	0	267	NA
Green Beans	1 order	124	6	2	NA	6	1843	NA
Macaroni & Cheese	1 order	241	14	8	NA		588	NA
Bread Service	1 order	263	7	1	NA	0	502	NA
Cranberry Sauce (1.5 oz.)	1 order	64	0	0	NA	0	12	NA
Breakfast Menu Selections								
All-Star Breakfast w/o options	1 order	190	15	7	NA	850	180	NA
Deluxe Pancake Platter	1 order	1609	32	6	NA	294	4988	NA
Half Stack Pancake Platter	1 order	932	14	3	NA	147	2592	NA
Big Eater Steak Breakfast w/o options	1 order	629	41	18	NA	1003	511	NA

Shoney's®
Continued

	Serving	Calories	Total fat (gm)	Saturated fat (gm)	Trans fats (gm)	Cholesterol (mg)	Sodium (mg)	Carbs (gm)
Breakfast Menu Selections continued								
Country Fried Steak Breakfast	1 order	994	66	20	NA	957	3594	NA
Sunrise Breakfast	1 order	973	60	16	NA	852	4001	NA
Sausage/Biscuit (1)	1 order	539	34	9	NA	48	1655	NA
Sausage/Biscuits (2)	1 order	1057	66	17	NA	96	3283	NA
Burgers								
A-A Bacon Cheeseburger	1 order	891	49	18	NA	195	1490	NA
All-American Burger	1 order	688	32	11	NA	150	932	NA
Mushroom Swiss Burger	1 order	969	58	19	NA	176	1122	NA
Famous Patty Melt	1 order	946	60	20	NA	190	1276	NA
Half-O-Pound Burger	1 order	1351	53	17	NA	225	1884	NA
Chicken								
Chicken Stir-Fry	1 order	1200	35	7	NA	103	4317	NA
Smothered Chicken	1 order	891	34	9	NA	125	2199	NA
Charbroiled Chicken Breast	1 order	797	23	4	NA	97	1831	NA
Charbroiled Blackened Chicken	1 order	831	26	4	NA	97	2017	NA
Fried Chicken Tenderloins	1 order	1157	61	8	NA	45	2514	NA
Monterey Chicken	1 order	909	40	9	NA	126	2067	NA
Desserts								
Ultimate Hot Fudge Cake	1 order	875	37	21	NA	99	784	NA
Original Strawberry Pie	1 slice	332	17	NA	NA	0	247	NA
Apple Pie a la Mode	1 order	1203	53	24	NA	49	1116	NA
Apple Pie w/ NutraSweet®	1 order	454	18	4	NA	0	415	NA
Cherry Pie w/ NutraSweet®	1 order	467	18	4	NA	0	441	NA
Peach Pie w/ NutraSweet®	1 order	479	21	4	NA	0	467	NA
Caramel Sundae	1 order	621	27	20	NA	88	332	NA
Hot Fudge Sundae	1 order	599	30	22	NA	80	228	NA
Strawberry Sundae	1 order	609	27	20	NA	88	189	NA
Walnut Brownie a la Mode	1 order	576	34	NA	NA	35	435	NA
Chocolate Milk Shake	1 order	1082	51	33	NA	190	531	NA
Strawberry Milk Shake	1 order	1115	50	33	NA	190	447	NA
Vanilla Milk Shake	1 order	1076	50	33	NA	190	432	NA
Cheesecake	1 slice	364	26	11	NA	62	188	NA
Junior Meals								
Junior Chicken	1 order	189	10	2	NA	27	532	NA
Junior Fish & Chips	1 order	308	11	2	NA	42	534	NA
Pasta								
Chicken Alfredo	1 order	1705	78	35	NA	427	3144	NA
Shrimp Alfredo	1 order	1781	85	39	NA	545	3243	NA

	Serving	Calories	Total fat (gm)	Saturated fat (gm)	Trans fats (gm)	Cholesterol (mg)	Sodium (mg)	Carbs (gm)
Pasta continued								
Italian Feast	1 order	1435	45	13	NA	262	4630	NA
Pasta Ya Ya	1 order	1847	81	32	NA	467	4738	NA
Items								
Raymond's French Dip	1 order	498	15	4	NA	76	2807	NA
Chicken Parmesan item	1 order	751	30	8	NA	99	2520	NA
Fried Chicken item	1 order	561	15	1	NA	67	3107	NA
Turkey Club	1 order	952	53	14	NA	178	2691	NA
Original Slim Jim	1 order	1004	34	9	NA	98	4392	NA
Ultimate Grilled Cheese	1 order	896	46	16	NA	102	2097	NA
Fish item	1 order	827	17	0	NA	67	2598	NA
Hot Roast Beef item w/ mashed potatoes & gravy	1 order	771	24	10	NA	98	2897	NA
Hot Turkey item w/ mashed potatoes & gravy	1 order	842	30	7	NA	79	1640	NA
Charbroiled Chicken item	1 order	894	22	2	NA	95	1914	NA
Blackened Chicken item	1 order	885	21	2	NA	95	2130	NA
Corned Beef Reuben	1 order	793	53	8	NA	179	4144	NA
Seafood								
Grilled Shrimp	1 order	720	19	3	NA	194	1401	NA
Grilled Salmon	1 order	749	19	3	NA	62	1623	NA
Shrimper's Feast	1 order	1032	39	5	NA	182	2131	NA
Shrimp Stir-Fry	1 order	873	19	4	NA	201	3975	NA
Fried Fish Platter	1 order	1049	39	5	NA	97	2047	NA
Fish 'n Shrimp	1 order	1098	39	5	NA	162	2155	NA
Steak								
Ribeye	8 oz.	1481	75	24	NA	189	2111	NA
Choice Sirloin	6 oz.	1224	51	14	NA	154	2073	NA
T-Bone	12 oz.	1809	100	33	NA	219	2187	NA
Half-O-Pound w/ grilled onions	1 order	1337	52	17	NA	225	1872	NA
Half-O-Pound w/ grilled mushrooms	1 order	1317	52	17	NA	225	3038	NA
Southwest Half-O-Pound	1 order	1304	69	23	NA	244	2943	NA
Surf & Turf								
Ribeye & 5 Fried Shrimp	1 order	1639	82	24	NA	284	2287	NA
Ribeye & 6 Grilled Shrimp	1 order	1589	81	25	NA	286	2258	NA
Sirloin & 5 Fried Shrimp	1 order	1382	58	14	NA	248	2249	NA
Sirloin & 6 Grilled Shrimp	1 order	1332	57	15	NA	250	2220	NA
T-Bone & 5 Fried Shrimp	1 order	1967	107	33	NA	313	2363	NA
T-Bone & 6 Grilled Shrimp	1 order	1918	106	34	NA	315	2334	NA
BBQ Ribs	1 order	1520	78	27	NA	NA	4033	NA

Shoney's®
Continued

Rib Combos (w/ fries)

	Serving	Calories	Total fat (gm)	Saturated fat (gm)	Trans fats (gm)	Cholesterol (mg)	Sodium (mg)	Carbs (gm)
¼ Rack & BBQ Chicken	1 order	1228	54	16	NA	95	3258	NA
¼ Rack & Tenderloins	1 order	1372	70	17	NA	47	3486	NA
¼ Rack & Fried Shrimp	1 order	1144	51	15	NA	88	2862	NA
¼ Rack & Grilled Shrimp	1 order	1125	53	15	NA	96	2808	NA
Miscellaneous								
Grilled Salmon, Lite	1 order	181	4	1	NA	60	152	NA
Grilled Cod, Lite	1 order	201	4	1	NA	94	402	NA
Grilled Shrimp, Lite	1 order	318	8	2	NA	194	585	NA

Fast Food Factoid:

People who regularly consume fruits, vegetables, whole grains, and nuts will have better health than those who do not; the data proves it.

Dr. Steven Aldana, The Culprit and The Cure

Sonic®
Breakfast

	Serving	Calories	Total fat (gm)	Saturated fat (gm)	Trans fats (gm)	Cholesterol (mg)	Sodium (mg)	Carbs (gm)
Bacon, Egg & Cheese Toaster	1 item	530	32	10	0.5	156	1698	40
Sausage, Egg & Cheese Toaster	1 item	620	42	13	1	126	1038	40
Ham, Egg & Cheese Toaster	1 item	490	26	8	0.5	174	2079	40
Breakfast Burrito	1 item	550	34	12	1.5	167	1535	38
Pancake on a Stick	3 oz.	240	14	7	NA	30	520	NA
Sunrise (regular)	18 fl. oz.	224	0	0	NA	0	41	NA
Hamburgers & Items								
Sonic Burger #1	1 item	650	37	10	1	37	753	54
Sonic Cheeseburger #1	1 item	720	42	14	1.5	52	1103	59
Bacon Cheeseburger	1 item	780	48	16	1.5	67	1433	57
Super Sonic #1	1 item	980	64	24	2.5	96	1476	60
Super Sonic #2	1 item	890	53	22	2.5	88	1571	NA
Country-Fried Steak item	1 item	748	47	12	NA	60	804	NA
Fish Sandwich	1 item	640	31	5	3	45	1180	71
Breaded Pork Fritter Sandwich	1 item	720	36	7	4	15	1010	66
Toaster Items								
BLT Toaster	1 item	581	41	9	NA	47	1307	NA
Bacon Cheddar Burger Toaster	1 item	670	39	14	1.5	59	1786	52
Chicken Club Toaster	1 item	740	46	11	0.5	85	1458	55

Toaster Items continued

	Serving	Calories	Total fat (gm)	Saturated fat (gm)	Trans fats (gm)	Cholesterol (mg)	Sodium (mg)	Carbs (gm)
Country-Fried Steak Toaster	1 item	708	45	11	NA	60	944	NA
Chicken								
Grilled Chicken item	1 item	343	13	2	0.5	70	829	32
Breaded Chicken item	1 item	582	23	4	0	53	427	49
Chicken Strip Dinner	1 meal	749	32	5	1	447	1973	100
Chicken Strip Snack	3 item	272	13	2	NA	35	760	NA
Jumbo Popcorn Chicken	4 oz.	347	20	4	0	44	1266	27
Salads								
Grilled Chicken Salad	1 salad	310	14	6	1	95	1050	19
Jumbo Popcorn Chicken Salad	1 salad	490	28	9	4	60	1440	39
Santa Fe Chicken Salad	1 salad	370	15	6	1	95	1140	29
Wraps								
Grilled Chicken Wrap w/ ranch dressing	1 wrap	539	27	5	NA	70	1035	NA
Grilled Chicken Wrap w/o ranch dressing	1 wrap	393	12	3	0	65	820	44
Chicken Strip Wrap w/ ranch dressing	1 wrap	574	29	5	NA	28	1071	NA
Chicken Strip Wrap w/o ranch dressing	1 wrap	428	13	2	0	23	856	54
Frito Chili Cheese Wrap	1 wrap	743	42	14	1	52	1172	66
Wacky Pack Kid's Meal (entrée only)								
Jr. Burger	1 item	353	21	6	0.5	45	1294	30
Hot Dog (plain)	1 item	262	16	5	NA	30	657	NA
Corn Dog	1 item	262	17	5	0	15	480	23
Grilled Cheese Toaster item	1 item	282	12	5	0.5	15	830	39
Chicken Strips	2 items	184	9	1	0	23	507	10
Coneys								
Coney (plain)	1 item	262	16	5	NA	30	657	NA
Corn Dog	1 item	210	11	3.5	0	20	530	23
Extra-Long Slaw Dog	1 item	670	38	12	1	80	1770	6
Extra-Long Chili Cheese Coney	1 item	600	33	11	1	75	1700	54
Faves & Craves Side Items								
French Fries (regular)	3.25 oz.	195	11	2	0	0	648	32
Cheese Fries (regular)	4.25 oz.	265	17	6	0	15	998	33
Chili Cheese Fries (regular)	5.25 oz.	299	19	6	0	22	952	35
Tator Tots (regular)	4.25 oz.	259	16	3	0	0	1046	24
Cheese Tots (regular)	5 oz.	329	22	7	0	15	1396	26
Chili Cheese Tater Tots (regular)	5.25 oz.	363	25	7	0.5	22	1350	27
Onion Rings (regular)	12.5 oz.	331	5	1	0	0	311	55

Sonic® Continued

Faves & Craves Side Items continued

	Serving	Calories	Total fat (gm)	Saturated fat (gm)	Trans fats (gm)	Cholesterol (mg)	Sodium (mg)	Carbs (gm)
Fritos Chili Pie	7 oz.	611	44	13	1	53	816	72
Mozzarella Sticks	5.5 oz.	382	19	11	0.5	50	1300	40
Ched'R' Peppers	4.5 oz.	256	12	5	1	28	1056	36
Burrito	1 item	370	20	7	1	15	520	40
Taco	1 item	310	18	6	2	25	370	35

Fast Food Factoid:
Even small increases in physical activity or fitness result in large improvements in health.

Starbucks®

Muffins & Scones

	Serving	Calories	Total fat (gm)	Saturated fat (gm)	Trans fats (gm)	Cholesterol (mg)	Sodium (mg)	Carbs (gm)
Blueberry Muffin	154 g	410	12	7	0	25	270	55
Blueberry Scone	142 g	500	29	18	0	100	330	64
Bran Muffin	156 g	420	19	2	0	45	470	NA
Carrot Walnut Muffin	154 g	540	24	2	0	0	330	NA
Cranberry Orange Muffin	1 item	460	24	8	0	100	580	NA
Chocolate Cream Cheese Muffin	153 g	600	43	11	0	0	220	NA
Cinnamon Chip Scone	128 g	540	29	19	0	90	80	NA
Low-Fat Blueberry Core Muffin	156 g	240	2	0	0	0	290	NA
Maple Oat Nut Scone	170 g	650	34	13	6	40	240	NA
Oat Nut Grain Muffin	137 g	490	23	11	0	60	360	NA
Pumpkin Cream Cheese Muffin	1 item	490	24	6	0	85	470	63
Pumpkin Scone	1 item	620	31	16	0	20	480	NA
Raspberry Scone	142 g	500	29	18	0	100	33	64
Triple Berry Cobbler Muffin	1 item	420	18	6	0	70	310	NA

Loaf Cakes & Coffee Cakes

	Serving	Calories	Total fat (gm)	Saturated fat (gm)	Trans fats (gm)	Cholesterol (mg)	Sodium (mg)	Carbs (gm)
Banana Loaf Cake (kosher wrapped)	113 g	360	18	11	0	100	380	56
No Sugar Added Banana Walnut Cake	1 item	360	21	3	0	20	330	NA
Carrott Cake Bar	1 item	390	25	8	0	60	380	NA
Crumble Coffee Cake (kosher wrapped)	163 g	670	32	15	1	115	360	NA
Cheese Twists	1 item	310	21	14	0	70	430	NA
Lemon Iced Pound Cake (kosher wrapped)	142 g	500	23	12	0	145	380	78
Marble Loaf (kosher wrapped)	113 g	400	21	11	0	130	370	52

Starbucks®
Continued

	Serving	Calories	Total fat (gm)	Saturated fat (gm)	Trans fats (gm)	Cholesterol (mg)	Sodium (mg)	Carbs (gm)
Loaf Cakes & Coffee Cakes continued								
Reduced-Fat Banana Bread	113 g	430	12	7	0	55	250	76
Reduced-Fat Blueberry Coffee Cake	124 g	350	11	6	1	10	430	54
Reduced-Fat Cinnamon Swirl Coffee Cake	105 g	330	8	5	1	5	400	52
Reduced-Fat Marble Coffee Cake	102 g	340	11	5	1	5	420	NA
Croissants, Bagels & Breads								
Asiago Focaccia Square	144 g	410	18	5	0	0	590	NA
Butter Croissant	99 g	440	25	16	0	70	200	NA
Chocolate Croissant	99 g	360	20	13	6	55	200	NA
Cinnamon Raisin Bagel	113 g	320	1	0	0	0	460	NA
Multigrain Bagel	113 g	360	4	0	0	0	480	60
Plain Bagel	113 g	320	1	0	0	0	480	62
Sesame Bagel	113 g	280	0	0	0	0	460	NA
Doughnuts, Sweet Rolls & Danish								
Almond Brioche Toast	102 g	360	17	6	0	20	250	NA
Apple Cinnamon Roll (fritter)	227 g	790	37	8	11	0	830	64
Cinnamon Sugar Cake Doughnut	99 g	400	19	4	6	20	420	NA
Glazed Doughnut	85 g	280	11	3	3	0	400	45
Brownies, Cookies & Bars								
Apple Cinnamon Bar	136 g	350	15	3	3	0	140	NA
Chocolate Chip Cookie	122 g	530	31	17	0	35	530	NA
Chocolate Petite Cookie	8 g	45	3	2	0	5	25	NA
Espresso Fudge Brownie	94 g	430	25	16	8	75	140	40
Gingerbread Petite Cookie	8 g	40	2	1	0	5	20	NA
Holiday Snowflake Cookie	78 g	340	16	6	2	20	170	NA
M & M Cookie	122 g	520	24	12	0	40	590	NA
Oatmeal Raisin Cookie	122 g	470	16	6	0	20	440	NA
Peppermint Petite Cookie	8 g	40	2	1	0	5	20	NA
Raspberry Petite Cookie	8 g	40	2	1	0	5	20	NA
Seven Layer Bar	133 g	600	37	17	3	10	270	NA
Snickerdoodle Cookie	75 g	310	14	7	0	25	240	13
Triple Chocolate Cookie	18 g	80	7	4	0	10	15	9
Toffee Almond Bar	94 g	430	21	7	4	50	440	53
Breakfast								
Black Forest Ham, Egg, & Cheddar	1 item	380	16	8	0	170	930	37
Classic Sausage, Egg, & Cheddar	1 item	470	25	11	0	185	850	37
Eggs Florentine w/ Baby Spinach & Havarti	1 item	390	19	10	0	168	780	NA

Starbucks®
Continued

Breakfast continued

	Serving	Calories	Total fat (gm)	Saturated fat (gm)	Trans fats (gm)	Cholesterol (mg)	Sodium (mg)	Carbs (gm)
Peppered Bacon, Egg, & Cheddar	1 item	390	18	9	0	160	850	37
Reduced Fat Turkey Bacon, Cholesterol-Free Egg, & Reduced-Fat White Cheddar	1 item	350	11	4	0	20	820	41

Beverages (size grande, whole milk where applicable)
Brewed Coffees

	Serving	Calories	Total fat (gm)	Saturated fat (gm)	Trans fats (gm)	Cholesterol (mg)	Sodium (mg)	Carbs (gm)
Coffee of the Week	16 oz.	10	0	0	0	0	0	0
Decaf Coffee of the Week	16 oz.	10	0	0	0	0	0	0
Iced Shaken Coffee	16 oz.	80	0	0	0	0	0	NA
Apple Juice	16 oz.	230	0	0	0	0	20	64
Blueberries & Cream Frappuccino Blended Crème-no whip	16 oz.	340	3	0	0	5	260	72
Blueberries & Cream Frappuccino Blended Crème- whip	16 oz.	470	15	8	0	55	270	74
Blueberries & Cream Frappuccino Blended Light Crème	16 oz.	190	1	0	0	5	150	45
Caffè Americano	16 oz.	15	0	0	0	0	0	3
Caffè Latte	16 oz.	260	14	9	0	55	200	18
Caffè Misto/Café Au Lait	16 oz.	140	8	5	0	30	115	9
Caffè Mocha w/o whip	16 oz.	300	12	6	0	30	135	40
Caffè Mocha w/ whip	16 oz.	400	22	13	0	80	160	42
Caffè Vanilla Frappuccino Blended Coffee w/o whip	16 oz.	340	4	2	0	15	260	67
Caffè Vanilla Frappuccino Blended Coffee w/ whip	16 oz.	470	16	10	0	65	270	70
Caffè Vanilla Frappuccino Light Blended Coffee w/o whip	16 oz.	230	1	0	0	5	310	NA
Caffè Vanilla Frappuccino Light Blended Coffee w/ whip	16 oz.	360	13	8	0	55	320	42
Cappuccino	16 oz.	150	8	5	0	30	115	11
Caramel Apple Cider w/o whip	16 oz.	300	0	0	0	0	15	NA
Caramel Apple Cider w/ whip	16 oz.	410	10	7	0	40	30	NA
Caramel Frappuccino Blended Coffee w/o whip	16 oz.	280	4	2	0	15	250	53
Caramel Frappuccino Blended Coffee w/ whip	16 oz.	430	16	10	0	65	270	57
Caramel Frappuccino Light Blended Coffee w/o whip	16 oz.	180	2	0	0	5	310	30
Caramel Frappuccino Light Blended Coffee w/ whip	16 oz.	310	14	8	0	55	320	NA
Caramel Macchiato	16 oz.	310	12	7	0	40	160	34
Chocolate Milk	16 oz.	340	15	8	0	50	190	51
Cinnamon Dolce Crème w/o whip	16 oz.	360	15	9	0	60	220	40
Cinnamon Dolce Crème w/ whip	16 oz.	470	24	15	0.5	100	220	41

Starbucks Continued Brewed Coffees continued	Serving	Calories	Total fat (gm)	Saturated fat (gm)	Trans fats (gm)	Cholesterol (mg)	Sodium (mg)	Carbs (gm)
Cinnamon Dolce Frappuccino Blended Coffee w/o whip	16 oz.	290	4	0	0	15	260	45
Cinnamon Dolce Frappuccino Blended Coffee w/ whip	16 oz.	420	16	10	0	65	270	55
Cinnamon Dolce Frappuccino Light Blended Coffee w/o whip	16 oz.	190	1	0	0	5	300	29
Cinnamon Dolce Frappuccino Light Blended Coffee w/ whip	16 oz.	320	13	8	0	55	310	NA
Cinnamon Dolce Latte w/o whip	16 oz.	340	13	8	0	50	190	39
Cinnamon Dolce Latte w/ whip	16 oz.	440	22	14	0.5	90	200	41
Cinnamon Spice Mocha w/o whip	16 oz.	330	12	7	0	45	170	NA
Cinnamon Spice Mocha w/ whip	16 oz.	430	22	14	0	85	180	NA
Coffee Frappuccino Blended Coffee	16 oz.	260	4	2	0	15	250	48
Coffee Frappuccino Light Blended Coffee w/o whip	16 oz.	150	1	0	0	5	300	25
Coffee Frappuccino Light Blended Coffee w/ whip	16 oz.	280	13	8	0	55	310	NA
Double Chocolate Chip Frappuccino Blended Crème w/o whip	16 oz.	460	12	6	0	5	400	75
Double Chocolate Chip Frappuccino Blended Crème w/ whip	16 oz.	590	24	14	0	55	410	78
Dulce de Leche Crème-no whip	16 oz.	400	11	6	0	40	350	63
Dulce de Leche Crème- whip	16 oz.	490	19	12	1	70	360	64
Dulce de Leche Frappuccino Blended Coffee-no whip	16 oz.	290	3	2	0	15	270	60
Dulce de Leche Frappuccino Blended Coffee-whip	16 oz.	420	15	10	0	65	290	62
Dulce de Leche Frappuccino Blended Crème-no whip	16 oz.	400	3	0	0	10	44	82
Dulce de Leche Frappuccino Blended Crème-whip	16 oz.	530	15	9	0	60	450	85
Dulce de Leche Light Blended Coffee	16 oz.	70	1	0	0	5	260	34
Dulce de Leche Latte-no whip	16 oz.	380	10	6	0	35	330	62
Dulce de Leche Latte-whip	16 oz.	470	17	11	1	65	340	64
Espresso Frappuccino Blended Coffee	16 oz.	230	3	2	0	10	220	38
Espresso Frappuccino Light Blended Coffee w/o whip	16 oz.	140	1	0	0	5	260	20
Espresso Frappuccino Light Blended Coffee w/ whip	16 oz.	270	13	8	0	55	270	NA
Hot Chocolate w/o whip	16 oz.	350	14	7	0	35	160	46
Hot Chocolate w/ whip	16 oz.	450	24	13	0.5	75	190	49
Iced Brewed Coffee	16 oz.	90	0	0	0	0	5	21

Starbucks®
Continued

Brewed Coffees continued

	Serving	Calories	Total fat (gm)	Saturated fat (gm)	Trans fats (gm)	Cholesterol (mg)	Sodium (mg)	Carbs (gm)
Iced Caffè Americano	16 oz.	15	0	0	0	0	0	3
Iced Caffè Latte	16 oz.	160	8	5	0	30	120	12
Iced Caffè Mocha w/o whip	16 oz.	220	8	4	0	25	95	38
Iced Caffè Mocha w/ whip	16 oz.	350	20	12	0.5	75	105	38
Iced Caramel Macchiato	16 oz.	270	10	6	0	40	150	33
Iced Caramel Mocha w/o whip	16 oz.	290	7	3	0	15	65	NA
Iced Caramel Mocha w/ whip	16 oz.	420	19	11	0	65	75	NA
Iced Dulce de Leche Latte-no whip	16 oz.	310	6	3	0	20	280	57
Iced Dulce de Leche Latte- whip	16 oz.	440	18	11	1	70	290	59
Iced Orange Mocha-no whip	16 oz.	280	7	3	0	15	70	54
Iced Orange Mocha-whip	16 oz.	400	18	10	0	55	80	58
Iced Pumpkin Spice Latte-no whip	16 oz.	270	6	4	0	20	160	43
Iced Pumpkin Spice Latte- whip	16 oz.	380	17	11	1	60	170	47
Iced Raspberry Mocha-no whip	16 oz.	290	7	3	0	18	60	57
Iced Raspberry Mocha-whip	16 oz.	410	18	10	1	55	70	60
Iced Sugar-Free Syrup Flavored Latte	16 oz.	130	6	4	0	20	105	11
Iced Shaken Coffee	16 oz.	80	0	0	0	0	5	NA
Iced Syrup-Flavored Latte	16 oz.	210	7	4	0	20	95	30
Iced Tazo Black Tea Latte	16 oz.	130	6	4	0	20	105	34
Iced Tazo Green Tea Latte	16 oz.	210	6	4	0	20	85	44
Iced Tazo Red Tea Latte	16 oz.	230	2	0	0	5	300	34
Iced Vanilla Latte	16 oz.	210	7	4	0	20	95	30
Iced White Chocolate Mocha w/o whip	16 oz.	360	11	8	0	25	210	55
Iced White Chocolate Mocha w/ whip	16 oz.	490	24	16	0.5	75	220	58
Java Chip Frappuccino Blended Coffee w/o whip	16 oz.	370	9	6	0	15	300	64
Java Chip Frappuccino Blended Coffee w/ whip	16 oz.	510	22	15	0	65	310	67
Java Chip Frappuccino Light Blended Coffee w/o whip	16 oz.	260	7	5	0	5	350	36
Java Chip Frappuccino Light Blended Coffee w/ whip	16 oz.	400	19	13	0.5	55	360	NA
Marble Mocha Macchiato	16 oz.	410	15	9	0	35	220	NA
Milk	16 oz.	270	15	9	0.5	60	220	24
Mocha Frappuccino Blended Coffee w/o whip	16 oz.	290	4	2	0	15	250	54
Mocha Frappuccino Blended Coffee w/ whip	16 oz.	420	16	10	0	65	260	57
Mocha Frappuccino Light Blended Coffee w/o whip	16 oz.	180	2	0	0	5	300	29

Starbucks®
Continued
Brewed Coffees continued

	Serving	Calories	Total fat (gm)	Saturated fat (gm)	Trans fats (gm)	Cholesterol (mg)	Sodium (mg)	Carbs (gm)
Mocha Frappuccino Light Blended Coffee w/ whip	16 oz.	310	14	8	0	55	310	29
Orange Crème Frappuccino Blended Crème-no whip	16 oz.	320	2	0	0	5	300	NA
Orange Crème Frappuccino Blended Coffee-whip	16 oz.	430	13	7	0	50	310	64
Orange Crème Frappuccino Light Blended Crème	16 oz.	140	0	0	0	5	160	67
Orange Mocha-no whip	16 oz.	360	11	5	0	25	120	32
Orange Mocha-whip	16 oz.	430	18	10	0	55	130	60
Orange Mocha Frappuccino Blended Coffee-no whip	16 oz.	270	4	2	0	10	220	62
Orange Mocha Frappuccino Blended Coffee-whip	16 oz.	390	15	9	0	55	230	56
Orange Mocha Frappuccino Light Blended Coffee	16 oz.	150	1	0	0	0	210	60
Pomegranate Frappuccion Juice Blend	16 oz.	240	0	0	0	0	10	32
Pumpkin Spice Crème-no whip	16 oz.	360	12	7	0	35	230	58
Pumpkin Spice Crème- whip	16 oz.	430	19	11	1	60	230	49
Pumpkin Spice Frappuccino Blended Coffee-no whip	16 oz.	290	4	2	0	15	260	51
Pumpkin Spice Frappuccino Blended Coffee-whip	16 oz.	400	15	9	0	55	280	59
Pumpkin Spice Frappuccino Blended Crème-no whip	16 oz.	360	3	0	0	5	350	62
Pumpkin Spice Frappuccino Blended Crème-whip	16 oz.	470	13	7	0	50	360	71
Pumpkin Spice Frappuccino Light Blended Crème	16 oz.	190	0	0	0	5	220	74
Pumpkin Spice Frappuccino Blended Coffee	16 oz.	150	1	0	0	0	240	42
Pumpkin Spice Latte-no whip	16 oz.	340	10	6	0	30	210	31
Pumpkin Spice Latte-whip	16 oz.	410	17	10	1	55	210	49
Raspberry Chocolate Frappuccino Blended Crème-no whip	16 oz.	320	3	1	0	5	230	51
Raspberry Chocolate Frappuccino Blended Crème- whip	16 oz.	430	14	7	0	45	240	66
Raspberry Chocolate Light Frappuccino Blended Crème	16 oz.	210	2	0	0	5	150	69
Raspberry Mocha-no whip	16 oz.	370	11	5	0	25	110	48
Raspberry Mocha-whip	16 oz.	440	18	10	1	55	120	65
Steamed Apple Cider	16 oz.	230	0	0	0	0	20	56
Steamed Milk	16 oz.	270	15	9	0	60	220	NA
Strawberries & Crème Frappuccino Blended Crème w/o whip	16 oz.	450	5	2	0	5	360	92

Starbucks®
Continued
Brewed Coffees continued

	Serving	Calories	Total fat (gm)	Saturated fat (gm)	Trans fats (gm)	Cholesterol (mg)	Sodium (mg)	Carbs (gm)
Strawberries & Crème Frappuccino Blended Crème w/ whip	16 oz.	580	17	10	0	55	370	95
Syrup-Flavored Latte	16 oz.	320	12	7	0	40	160	36
Tazo Black Iced Tea	16 oz.	80	0	0	0	0	10	21
Tazo Black Tea Lemonade	16 oz.	120	0	0	0	0	15	33
Tazo Chai Crème Frappuccino Blended Tea w/o whip	16 oz.	380	5	2	0	5	360	67
Tazo Chai Crème Frappuccino Blended Tea w/ whip	16 oz.	510	17	10	0	55	370	71
Tazo Chai Iced Tea Latte	16 oz.	270	7	4	0	25	110	44
Tazo Chai Tea Latte	16 oz.	290	7	5	0	30	120	43
Tazo Green Iced Tea	16 oz.	80	0	0	0	0	10	21
Tazo Green Tea Frappuccino Blended Crème with Melon Syrup w/o whip	16 oz.	370	5	2	0	5	380	78
Tazo Green Tea Frappuccino Blended Crème with Melon Syrup w/ whip	16 oz.	500	16	9	0	60	390	82
Tazo Green Tea Lemonade	16 oz.	120	0	0	0	0	15	NA
Tazo Passion Iced Tea	16 oz.	80	0	0	0	0	10	19
Tazo Passion Tea Lemonade	16 oz.	120	0	0	0	0	15	NA
Toffee Nut Crème w/o whip	16 oz.	350	15	9	0	60	370	NA
Toffee Nut Crème w/ whip	16 oz.	450	24	15	0	100	380	NA
Toffee Nut Frappuccino Crème w/o whip	16 oz.	360	5	1	0	5	490	NA
Toffee Nut Frappuccino Crème w/ whip	16 oz.	480	17	9	0	55	500	NA
Toffee Nut Latte w/o whip	16 oz.	330	13	8	0	50	340	NA
Toffee Nut Latte w/ whip	16 oz.	420	22	14	0	90	350	NA
Vanilla Bean Frappuccino Blended Crème w/o whip	16 oz.	370	5	2	0	5	360	72
Vanilla Bean Frappuccino Blended Crème w/ whip	16 oz.	500	17	10	0	55	370	75
Vanilla Crème w/o whip	16 oz.	330	14	8	0	40	180	36
Vanilla Crème w/ whip	16 oz.	440	23	14	0.5	80	190	38
Vanilla Latte	16 oz.	320	12	7	0	40	160	36
White Chocolate Frappuccino Blended Crème w/o whip	16 oz.	480	9	5	0	10	470	89
White Chocolate Frappuccino Blended Crème w/ whip	16 oz.	610	21	13	0	60	480	92
White Chocolate Mocha w/o whip	16 oz.	410	15	10	0	45	250	60
White Chocolate Mocha w/ whip	16 oz.	510	24	16	0.5	80	260	62
White Chocolate Mocha Frappuccino Blended Coffee w/o whip	16 oz.	320	5	3	0	15	280	59

Starbucks®
Continued
Brewed Coffees continued

	Serving	Calories	Total fat (gm)	Saturated fat (gm)	Trans fats (gm)	Cholesterol (mg)	Sodium (mg)	Carbs (gm)
White Chocolate Mocha Frappuccino Blended Coffee w/ whip	16 oz.	450	17	11	0	65	290	62
White Chocolate Mocha Frappuccino Light Blended Coffee w/o whip	16 oz.	200	3	1	0	5	330	34
White Chocolate Mocha Frappuccino Light Blended Coffee w/ whip	16 oz.	340	15	9	0	55	340	NA
White Hot Chocolate w/o whip	16 oz.	480	18	12	0	55	300	61

Steak 'n Shake®
Breakfast

	Serving	Calories	Total fat (gm)	Saturated fat (gm)	Trans fats (gm)	Cholesterol (mg)	Sodium (mg)	Carbs (gm)
Eggs With the Works-Bacon	1 meal	876	70	17	NA	478	1241	NA
Eggs With the Works-Sausage	1 meal	1076	90	26	NA	518	1361	NA
Steak 'n Eggs Breakfast	1 meal	1016	80	22	NA	536	811	NA
Just Biscuits 'n Gravy	1 order	1311	75	28.5	20	70	3900	117
Biscuits, Gravy 'n Hash Browns	1 order	1567	91	32	24	100	4425	143
Strawberry French Toast	3 slices	467	12	4.5	0.5	98	329	81
Classic Stack 'o Cakes	1 order	375	18	3.5	2	12	915	47
The Strawberry Stack	1 order	586	23	6.5	2	25	924	NA
Cakes 'n Eggs 'n Bacon 'n Sausage	1 meal	764	58	18	NA	480	1296	NA
Country Scrambler	1 meal	925	67.5	22	6.5	567	2068	42
Cheddar Scrambler	1 meal	1149	80	21.5	10	562	2315	72

Breakfast Items

	Serving	Calories	Total fat (gm)	Saturated fat (gm)	Trans fats (gm)	Cholesterol (mg)	Sodium (mg)	Carbs (gm)
Steak, Egg & Cheese	1 item	546	35	13	NA	273	929	NA
Egg, Cheese & Sausage	1 item	576	40	15	NA	263	1204	NA
Egg, Cheese & Bacon	1 item	476	30	10	NA	243	1144	NA
Egg & Cheese	1 item	366	20	7	NA	228	894	NA
Sausage & Biscuit	1 item	638	44	13	NA	35	650	NA

Breakfast Side Items

	Serving	Calories	Total fat (gm)	Saturated fat (gm)	Trans fats (gm)	Cholesterol (mg)	Sodium (mg)	Carbs (gm)
One Egg, cooked w/ margarine	1 egg	119	10	2.5	0.5	211	70	0
Cholesterol-Free Scrambled Eggs	2 eggs	158	10	2	1.5	0	181	2
Bacon	4 strips	196	14	5	0	445	685	2
Sausage Patties	2 items	432	40	14	0	84	714	2
Sausage Gravy	5 oz.	256	18.5	9.5	0	35	720	12
Buttermilk Pancakes	2 items	250	12	2	1.5	8	610	31
Cinnamon Swirl French Toast	3 slices	256	7	1.5	0.5	85	320	40
Hash Browns	1 order	256	16	3.5	4.5	30	525	25

Steak 'n Shake®
Continued

	Serving	Calories	Total fat (gm)	Saturated fat (gm)	Trans fats (gm)	Cholesterol (mg)	Sodium (mg)	Carbs (gm)
Breakfast Side Items continued								
Buttermilk Biscuit w/o margarine	1 item	400	19	5	10	0	1230	47
English Muffin w/o margarine	1 item	140	1.5	0	0	0	300	27
Bagel (plain)	1 item	320	2	0	0	0	600	67
Steakburgers								
Original Single	1 item	250	9.5	3.5	0.5	35	385	26
Original Single w/ cheese	1 item	310	14.5	6.5	0.5	45	585	26
Original Double	1 item	350	15.5	6	1	70	420	26
Original Double w/ cheese	1 item	410	20.5	9	1	80	620	26
Bacon 'n Cheese Double	1 item	508	27.5	11.5	1	103	962	27
Deluxe Cheddar 'n Bacon	1 item	809	49	18	NA	115	1304	39
Mushroom 'n Swiss	1 item	586	29	13.5	1	110	725	38
The Philadelphia	1 item	594	31.5	9.5	4	79	950	44
The BBQ 'n Bacon	1 item	875	49	20	NA	128	1385	46
Triple Steakburger Sandwich	1 item	450	21.5	8.5	1.5	105	455	NA
Triple Steakburger Sandwich w/ Cheese	1 item	570	31.5	14.5	1.5	125	855	NA
Cheddar 'n Bacon Steakburger	1 item	572	28	10.5	2.5	102	1292	39
Grilled Mushroom & Onion Steakburger	1 item	504	23	9	1	80	1135	NA
Hickory Smoked Thick Bacon Steakburger	1 item	610	30	12	1	112	1375	39
BBQ Ranch premium Steakburger	1 item	633	31	10	1	107	1613	46
Portobello & Swiss Steakburger	1 item	512	21	9	1	91	843	41
Black Peppercorn Bacon Steakburger	1 item	620	31	13	1	112	1395	40
Melts								
Frisco Melt	1 item	980	72	20	5	115	1199	42
Patty Melt	1 item	810	61	17.5	6	90	870	30
Chicken Melt	1 item	936	64	14.5	4	130	2025	46
Pepperjack Melt	1 item	958	73	20.5	6.5	100	1002	39
Turkey Melt	1 item	950	70	16	NA	98	1928	47
Tuna Melt	1 item	919	77	18	NA	87	1873	NA
Specialty Items								
Spicy Chicken item	1 item	542	32	5	0.5	40	1551	56
Grilled Chicken Breast	1 item	471	26	4	NA	52	726	NA
Bacon, Lettuce 'n Tomato	1 item	528	34	9	0	440	974	43
Chicken Fingers 'n Fries	1 item	508	31	5	2	23	342	45
Grilled Cheese	1 item	680	51	17	5	45	1450	40
Grilled Cheese 'n Bacon	1 item	790	61	20	5	60	1700	41
Tuna Salad	1 item	445	30	4	NA	48	1021	NA

Steak 'n Shake®
Continued
Specialty Items continued

	Serving	Calories	Total fat (gm)	Saturated fat (gm)	Trans fats (gm)	Cholesterol (mg)	Sodium (mg)	Carbs (gm)
Fish Fillet item	1 item	398	17	3.5	0.5	58	1105	43
Turkey Club	1 item	576	35	8	0	77	1521	46
Salads w/ dressing								
Fried Chicken Salad	1 salad	698	53	18	0	101	931	20
Chicken Chef Salad	1 salad	463	32	12	NA	92	654	NA
Deluxe Garden Salad	1 salad	226	15	9	NA	45	312	17
Beef Taco Salad	1 salad	940	59	17	NA	71	1876	66
Chicken Taco Salad	1 salad	1072	70	17	NA	100	1839	64
Garden Salad, small	1 salad	198	11	4.5	0	25	359	NA
Apple Walnut Grilled Chicken Salad	1 salad	337	10	0	0	72	804	38
Classic Grilled Chicken Salad	1 salad	466	25	8	0	120	1675	23
Apples & Grapes w/ Caramel Dip	1 item	285	3	2	0	11	200	NA
Chili								
Genuine Chili	6 oz.	389	26	10	0	64	1120	17
Chili Deluxe	6 oz.	538	38	17	0.5	102	1319	21
Chili Mac	1 order	696	30	14	NA	37	1176	89
Chili 3-Way	1 order	823	45	17.5	0	108	2048	65
Chili 5-Way	1 order	1120	69	31	1.5	184	2445	74
Side Items								
French Fries (small)	2.25 oz.	260	12	3	1	0	288	31
Cheddar Cheese Fries (small)	2.25 oz.	336	19	6	2.5	10	749	34
Onion Rings (small)	4.5 oz.	334	20	3	1	0	714	41
Creamy Coleslaw	3.5 oz.	306	24	4	0	45	411	20
Old-Fashioned Baked Beans	1 Crock	372	1	0	0	0	1466	74
Vegetable Beef Soup	6 oz.	60	2	0	0	0	680	12
Chicken Noodle Soup	6 oz.	80	2	1	0	5	690	10
Broccoli Cheese Soup	6 oz.	90	5	3	1	10	830	10
Chicken Gumbo Soup	6 oz.	80	2	1	0	10	880	14

NOTES:

_____

_____

_____

_____

Subway®

	Serving	Calories	Total fat (gm)	Saturated fat (gm)	Trans fats (gm)	Cholesterol (mg)	Sodium (mg)	Carbs (gm)
6" Items with 6 Grams of Fat or Less								
Honey Mustard Ham	1 item	320	5	2	0	25	1420	47
Oven-Roasted Chicken Breast	1 item	330	5	2	0	45	1020	48
Roast Beef	1 item	290	5	2	0	20	920	45
Savory Turkey Breast	1 item	280	5	2	0	20	1020	46
Savory Turkey Breast & Ham	1 item	290	5	2	0	25	1230	47
Subway Club	1 item	320	6	2	0	35	1310	47
Sweet Onion Chicken Teriyaki	1 item	370	5	2	0	50	1220	59
Veggie Delite	1 item	230	3	1	0	0	520	44
6" Fresh Toasted Items								
Cheese Steak	1 item	360	10	5	0	35	1090	NA
Chipotle Southwest Cheese Steak	1 item	450	20	6	0	45	1310	NA
Italian BMT	1 item	450	21	8	0	55	1790	NA
Meatball Marinara	1 item	560	24	11	1	45	1610	NA
Turkey Breast, Ham & Bacon Melt	1 item	380	12	5	0	45	1610	NA
Chicken Bacon Ranch	1 item	530	25	10	0	90	1400	NA
6" Cold Items								
Classic Tuna	1 item	530	31	7	1	45	1030	44
Cold Cut Combo	1 item	410	17	7	1	60	1550	47
Subway Seafood Sensation (processsed seafood & crab blend)	1 item	450	22	6	1	25	1150	NA
Deli-Style Items								
BBQ Rib Patty	1 item	420	19	6	0	50	810	NA
BBQ Chicken	1 item	310	6	2	0	35	1090	NA
Buffalo Chicken	1 item	380	18	4	0	55	1490	NA
Gardenburger	1 item	390	7	3	0	5	950	NA
Classic Tuna	1 item	350	18	5	1	30	750	NA
Ham	1 item	210	4	2	0	10	770	NA
Roast Beef	1 item	220	5	2	0	15	660	NA
Savory Turkey Breast	1 item	210	4	2	0	15	730	NA
Veggy Patty	1 item	390	8	2	0	10	1080	NA
8" Pizza								
Cheese	1 pizza	680	22	9	0	40	1070	96
Cheese & Veggies	1 pizza	740	25	11	0	50	1210	100
Pepperoni	1 pizza	790	32	13	0	60	1350	96
Sausage	1 pizza	830	35	14	0	71	1450	97
Breakfast Sandwiches on 6" Bread								
Cheese	1 item	400	17	7	0	160	940	43
Chipotle Steak & Cheese	1 item	580	31	11	1	200	1400	48

Subway® Continued

	Serving	Calories	Total fat (gm)	Saturated fat (gm)	Trans fats (gm)	Cholesterol (mg)	Sodium (mg)	Carbs (gm)
Breakfast Sandwiches on 6" Bread continued								
Double Bacon & Cheese	1 item	500	25	11	1	180	1310	44
Honey Mustard Ham & Cheese	1 item	460	19	8	0	175	1430	51
Western w/ Cheese	1 item	440	18	8	0	175	1320	45
Wraps								
Chicken & Bacon Ranch w/ cheese	1 wrap	440	27	10	0	90	1670	NA
Tuna w/ cheese	1 wrap	440	32	6	1	45	1310	NA
Turkey Breast	1 wrap	190	6	1	0	20	1290	NA
Turkey Breast & Bacon Melt w/ chipotle sauce	1 wrap	440	28	10	0	65	1870	NA
Salads (w/o dressing or croutons)								
Grilled Chicken & Baby Spinach	1 salad	140	3	1	0	50	450	NA
Subway Club	1 salad	160	4	2	0	35	880	NA
Tuna w/ cheese	1 salad	360	29	6	1	45	600	NA
Veggie Delite	1 salad	60	1	0	0	0	90	NA
Jared Salads w/ 6g of Fat or Less								
Ham	1 salad	120	3	1	0	25	840	14
Oven Roasted Chicken Breast	1 salad	140	3	1	0	50	390	11
Roast Beef	1 salad	120	3	2	0	20	480	12
Sweet Onion Chicken Teriyaki	1 salad	210	3	1	0	50	780	26
Turkey Breast	1 salad	110	3	1	0	20	580	13
Turkey Breast & Ham	1 salad	120	3	1	0	25	790	14
Veggie Delite	1 salad	60	1	0	0	0	80	11
Breads								
Italian (white)	6 Inch	200	3	2	0	0	340	38
Wheat	6 Inch	200	3	1	0	0	360	40
Italian Herbs & Cheese	6 Inch	240	6	3	0	8	540	40
Honey Oat	6 Inch	250	4	1	0	0	380	48
Parmesan Oregano	6 Inch	210	4	2	0	0	500	40
Hearty Italian	6 Inch	210	3	2	0	0	340	41
Monterey Cheddar	6 Inch	240	6	4	0	10	400	39
Deli-Style Roll	1 roll	170	3	1	0	0	280	NA
Carb Concious Wrap	1 wrap	120	5	0	0	0	680	NA
Cheese (standard amounts for 6" subs, wraps, or salads)								
Processed American	.5 oz.	40	4	2	0	10	200	1
Shredded Monterey Cheddar	1 oz.	110	9	6	0	30	180	1
Natural Cheddar	.5 oz.	60	5	3	0	15	95	0
Pepperjack	.5 oz.	50	4	3	0	15	140	0
Provolone	.5 oz.	50	4	2	0	10	125	0
Swiss	.5 oz.	50	5	3	0	15	30	0

Subway® Continued

Soups

	Serving	Calories	Total fat (gm)	Saturated fat (gm)	Trans fats (gm)	Cholesterol (mg)	Sodium (mg)	Carbs (gm)
Chicken Dumpling	10 oz	170	5	2	0	35	1390	23
Chili con Carne	10 oz	290	8	4	0	25	990	35
Cream of Broccoli	10 oz	160	7	3	0	10	1010	18
Cream of Potato w/ Bacon	10 oz	240	13	5	0	15	1050	26
Golden Broccoli & Cheese	10 oz	200	12	5	0	25	1180	17
Minestrone	10 oz	80	1	1	0	<5	1125	15
New England Clam Chowder	10 oz	150	5	1	0	10	990	20
Roasted Chicken Noodle	10 oz	80	2	1	0	15	240	11
Spanish Style Chicken w/ Rice	10 oz	110	2	1	0	10	1300	17
Tomato Garden Vegetable w/ Rotini	10 oz	90	0	0	0	0	1140	20
Vegetable Beef	10 oz	100	2	1	0	0	1450	15
Wild Rice w/ Chicken	10 oz	210	11	4	0	25	1250	21

Taco Bell®

Tacos

	Serving	Calories	Total fat (gm)	Saturated fat (gm)	Trans fats (gm)	Cholesterol (mg)	Sodium (mg)	Carbs (gm)
Taco	1 taco	170	10	4	1	25	350	13
Spicy Chicken Taco	1 taco	180	7	2	1	20	580	20
Taco Supreme	1 taco	220	14	7	1	35	360	15
Soft Taco (beef)	1 taco	210	10	4	1	25	620	21
Double Decker Taco	1 taco	340	14	5	2	25	810	38
Double Decker Taco Supreme	1 taco	380	18	8	2	40	820	40
Ranchero Chicken Soft Taco	1 taco	270	14	4	1	35	710	21
Grilled Steak Soft Taco	1 taco	280	17	5	1	30	650	NA
Grande Soft Taco	1 taco	450	21	8	3	45	1410	43
Soft Taco Supreme (beef)	1 taco	260	14	7	1	35	640	23

Burritos

	Serving	Calories	Total fat (gm)	Saturated fat (gm)	Trans fats (gm)	Cholesterol (mg)	Sodium (mg)	Carbs (gm)
Bean Burrito	1 item	370	10	4	2	10	1200	54
7-Layer Burrito	1 item	530	21	8	3	25	1350	65
Chili Cheese Burrito	1 item	390	18	9	2	40	1080	NA
Spicy Chicken Burrito	1 item	430	19	5	2	30	1160	48
Burrito Supreme (beef)	1 item	440	18	8	2	40	1330	51
Burrito Supreme (chicken)	1 item	410	14	6	2	45	1270	49
Burrito Supreme (steak)	1 item	420	16	7	2	35	1260	49
Grilled Stuffed Burrito (beef)	1 item	720	33	11	4	55	2090	76
Grilled Stuffed Burrito (chicken)	1 item	680	26	7	3	70	1950	73
Grilled Stuffed Burrito (steak)	1 item	680	28	8	3	55	1940	72
Fiesta Burrito (beef)	1 item	390	15	5	2	25	1160	49

Burritos continued

	Serving	Calories	Total fat (gm)	Saturated fat (gm)	Trans fats (gm)	Cholesterol (mg)	Sodium (mg)	Carbs (gm)
Fiesta Burrito (chicken)	1 item	370	12	4	2	30	1090	47
Fiesta Burrito (steak)	1 item	370	13	4	2	25	1080	47
Gorditas								
Nacho Cheese (beef)	1 order	300	13	4	2	20	740	31
Nacho Cheese (chicken)	1 order	270	10	3	1	25	670	29
Nacho Cheese (steak)	1 order	270	11	3	2	20	660	29
Supreme (beef)	1 order	310	16	7	1	35	600	29
Supreme (chicken)	1 order	290	12	5	0	45	530	28
Supreme (steak)	1 order	290	13	6	1	35	520	28
Baja (beef)	1 order	350	19	5	1	30	760	29
Baja (chicken)	1 order	320	15	4	0	40	690	28
Baja (steak)	1 order	320	16	4	0	30	680	27
Chalupas								
Nacho Cheese (beef)	1 order	380	22	7	4	20	740	32
Nacho Cheese (chicken)	1 order	350	18	5	4	25	670	30
Nacho Cheese (steak)	1 order	350	19	5	4	20	670	30
Supreme (beef)	1 order	390	24	10	3	35	600	30
Supreme (chicken)	1 order	370	20	8	3	45	530	29
Supreme (steak)	1 order	370	22	8	3	35	520	28
Baja (beef)	1 order	430	27	8	3	30	760	30
Baja (chicken)	1 order	440	24	6	3	40	690	29
Baja (steak)	1 order	400	25	7	3	30	680	28
Specialties								
Tostada	1 item	250	10	4	2	15	710	NA
Crunchwrap Supreme	1 item	560	24	8	2	35	1430	68
Grilled Steak Taquitos	1 item	320	11	5	0	35	1030	NA
Spicy Chickenwrap Supreme	1 item	540	23	7	2	40	1360	67
Mexican Pizza	1 pizza	550	31	11	5	45	1040	46
Meximelt	1 item	290	16	8	1	40	880	22
Enchirito (beef)	1 order	380	18	9	2	45	1430	34
Enchirito (chicken)	1 order	350	14	7	2	55	1360	33
Enchirito (steak)	1 order	360	16	8	2	45	1350	33
Cheese Quesadilla	1 item	490	28	13	2	55	1150	NA
Chicken Quesadilla	1 item	540	30	13	2	80	1380	40
Steak Quesadilla	1 item	540	31	14	2	70	1370	39
Fresco Style								
Crunchy Taco	1 taco	150	7	3	1	20	360	NA
Rancho Chicken Soft Taco	1 taco	170	4	1	1	25	710	NA
Grilled Steak Soft Taco	1 taco	170	5	2	1	15	560	NA

Taco Bell®
Continued

Fresco Style continued

	Serving	Calories	Total fat (gm)	Saturated fat (gm)	Trans fats (gm)	Cholesterol (mg)	Sodium (mg)	Carbs (gm)
Gordita Baja (chicken)	1 order	230	6	1	0	25	570	NA
Gordita Baja (steak)	1 order	230	7	2	0	15	570	NA
Tostada	1 item	200	6	1	1	0	670	NA
Enchirito (chicken)	1 order	250	5	2	1	25	1230	NA
Bowls & Salads								
Southwest Steak Bowl w/ dressing	1 salad	700	32	8	4	55	2050	68
Zesty Chicken Border Bowl w/ dressing	1 salad	730	42	9	4	45	1640	60
Fiesta Taco Salad w/ salsa	1 salad	870	47	16	9	65	1780	80
Fiesta Taco Salad w/ salsa w/o shell or strips	1 salad	420	21	10	2	65	1480	41
Express Taco Salad w/ chips	1 salad	630	33	13	5	65	1390	56
Express taco Salad w/o chips	1 salad	410	21	10	2	65	1300	NA
Nachos & Sides								
Cheesy Fiesta Potatoes	5 oz.	280	18	6	4	20	800	30
Nachos	3.5 oz	320	19	5	5	5	530	32
Nachos Supreme	7 oz.	450	26	9	5	35	810	41
Nachos BellGrande	11 oz.	780	43	13	10	35	1300	77
Mexican Rice	4.75 oz	210	10	4	2	15	740	23
Pintos 'n Cheese	4.5 oz	180	7	4	1	15	700	19
Cinnamon Twists	1.25 oz	160	5	1	2	0	150	26

Fast Food Factoid:

Of all the restaurants in this guide, Panda Express is ranked number one in promoting public health. No trans fats are used at Panda Express and most items include fresh vegetables.

NOTES:

_____

_____

_____

_____

_____

_____

_____

_____

Taco John's®

	Serving	Calories	Total fat (gm)	Saturated fat (gm)	Trans fats (gm)	Cholesterol (mg)	Sodium (mg)	Carbs (gm)
Tacos								
Taco Bravo	1 taco	340	14	5	2	25	650	39
Beefy Cheesy Taco Bravo	1 taco	410	22	9	NA	50	850	NA
Crispy Taco	1 taco	180	10	4	0	25	270	13
Softshell Taco	1 taco	220	10	5	1	25	470	21
Chicken Softshell Taco	1 taco	190	6	3	1	30	760	19
Low-Carb Beef Softshell Taco	1 taco	190	10	4	NA	25	520	NA
Low-Carb Chicken Softshell Taco	1 taco	160	6	3	NA	30	800	NA
El Grande Taco	1 taco	510	32	11	NA	75	820	NA
El Grande Chicken Taco	1 taco	380	20	7	NA	60	1010	NA
Beef Taco in a Bag	1 taco	180	12	6	NA	40	420	NA
Chicken Taco in a Bag	1 taco	140	7	4	NA	50	790	NA
Taco Burger	1 item	280	12	5	0	35	600	28
Burritos								
Bean Burrito	1 item	380	12	5	2	15	830	53
Beefy Burrito	1 item	430	20	9	1	55	870	41
Beef Grilled Burrito	1 item	590	32	15	2	75	1240	49
Chicken Grilled Burrito	1 item	590	30	13	1	95	1790	47
Chicken Festiva Burrito	1 item	530	24	7	NA	50	1300	NA
Chicken Fajita Burrito	1 item	340	11	5	NA	50	1120	NA
Chicken & Potato Burrito	1 item	460	19	7	3	35	1470	54
Crunchy Chicken & Potato Burrito	1 item	590	29	8	3	35	1420	62
Meat & Potato Burrito	1 item	490	23	8	4	30	1190	55
El Grande Burrito	1 item	720	36	17	NA	90	1640	NA
El Grande Chicken Burrito	1 item	660	28	13	NA	100	2210	NA
Ranch Burrito (beef)	1 item	420	22	7	NA	45	860	41
Ranch Burrito (chicken)	1 item	390	18	6	NA	50	1140	40
Combination Burrito	1 item	400	16	7	2	35	850	47
Steak Grilled Burrito	1 item	600	35	20	1	55	1020	46
Steak & Potato Burrito	1 item	590	30	15	3	35	1420	53
Steak & Rice Burrito	1 item	520	20	15	0	15	1040	67
Super Burrito	1 item	450	20	9	NA	40	920	49
Smothered Burrito	1 item	500	21	10	NA	50	1330	55
Specialties								
Chilito	1 order	430	22	12	NA	60	1040	NA
Chili Enchilada	1 item	740	38	12	NA	75	1470	24
Double Enchilada	1 item	720	40	18	NA	105	2090	NA
Tostada	1 item	180	10	4	NA	25	270	NA
Bean Tostada	1 item	160	6	2	NA	5	250	NA
Cheese Quesadilla	1 item	480	28	15	NA	50	960	39

Taco John's®
Continued

Specialties continued

	Serving	Calories	Total fat (gm)	Saturated fat (gm)	Trans fats (gm)	Cholesterol (mg)	Sodium (mg)	Carbs (gm)
Chicken Quesadilla	1 item	540	29	15	NA	75	1430	41
Mexi Rolls	7.5 oz	480	30	10	1	50	1270	NA
Mexi Rolls w/o nacho cheese	4.5 oz	370	21	6	NA	40	530	35

Platters

Beef Enchilada Platter	1 meal	780	37	15	NA	70	2460	NA
Chicken Enchilada Platter	1 meal	700	32	13	NA	65	2460	NA
Beef & Bean Chimi Platter	1 meal	760	34	11	NA	50	1930	NA
Smothered Burrito Platter	1 meal	830	33	13	NA	55	2230	NA

Salads (w/o dressing)

Side Salad	1 salad	80	5	2	0	5	50	6
Chicken Festiva Salad	1 salad	580	24	10	0	65	1190	24
Crunchy Chicken Festiva Salad	1 salad	750	37	11	0	60	1140	35
Taco Salad	1 salad	580	32	13	0	60	960	46
Chicken Taco Salad	1 salad	530	27	11	0	70	1330	44

Salad Dressings & Dipping Sauces

House Salad Dressing	2 oz.	90	10	2	0	0	360	3
Creamy Italian Salad Dressing	2 oz.	180	20	3	0	0	430	3
Ranch Salad Dressing	2 oz.	190	21	3	0	30	470	3
Bacon Ranch Salad Dressing	2 oz.	170	13	2	0	15	490	10
Chipotle Cream Sauce	2 oz.	300	30	6	0	20	380	4
Barbeque Dipping Sauce	1.25 oz.	50	0	0	0	0	340	NA
Honey Mustard Dipping Sauce	1.25 oz.	170	15	3	0	5	180	NA
Sweet & Sour Dipping Sauce	1.25 oz.	60	0	0	0	0	140	NA

Side Items

Cheese Crisp	2 oz.	210	14	7	NA	35	260	NA
Potato Olés (small)	5.25 oz.	440	26	6	9	0	1270	48
Super Potato Olés	16 oz.	980	62	22	15	60	2950	91
Potato Olés Bravo	8.25 oz.	580	36	11	8	20	1760	NA
Chili Potato Olés	11 oz.	610	36	11	NA	25	2290	59
Nachos	5 oz.	380	23	6	0	10	970	38
Super Nachos	12.75 oz.	830	51	17	1	60	1730	73
Chicken Super Nachos	12.25 oz.	780	45	15	1	90	2250	62
Refried Beans	9.5 oz.	400	14	5	4	15	1110	50
Mexican Rice	6 oz.	240	8	2	1	0	850	45
Texas-Style Chili	8.5 oz.	270	12	6	1	35	1400	26
Churro	1 order	235	10	2	3	10	120	31
Appe Grande	1 order	240	10	3	0	5	230	48
Choco Taco	1 order	385	20	15	0	15	161	41

Texas Roadhouse®

	Serving	Calories	Total fat (gm)	Saturated fat (gm)	Trans fats (gm)	Cholesterol (mg)	Sodium (mg)	Carbs (gm)

Does not provide nutrition information.

T.G.I. Friday's®
Does not provide nutrition information.

Waffle House®
Does not provide nutrition information.

Wendy's®

Items

	Serving	Calories	Total fat (gm)	Saturated fat (gm)	Trans fats (gm)	Cholesterol (mg)	Sodium (mg)	Carbs (gm)
Jr. Hamburger	1 item	280	9	4	0.5	30	600	26
Jr. Cheeseburger	1 item	320	13	6	0.5	40	810	26
Jr. Cheeseburger Deluxe	1 item	360	16	6	0.5	45	880	28
Jr. Bacon Cheeseburger	1 item	380	18	7	0.5	55	810	26
Hamburger (Kid's Meal)	1 item	270	9	4	0.5	30	600	25
Cheeseburger (Kid's Meal)	1 item	320	13	6	0.5	40	810	26
Classic Single w/ everything	1 item	430	20	7	1	65	890	37
Big Bacon Classic	1 item	580	29	12	1.5	95	1390	NA
Ultimate Chicken Grill item	1 item	360	7	2	0	75	1090	36
Spicy Chicken Fillet item	1 item	510	19	4	0	55	1480	46
Homestyle Chicken Fillet	1 item	540	22	4	0	55	1320	48
Ham & Cheese Sandwich (kids meal)	1 item	200	5	3	0	30	810	25
Turkey & Cheese Sandwich (Kids Meal)	1 item	210	6	3	0	25	830	27
Baconator	1 item	830	51	22	3	170	1920	35
Chicken Club Sandwich	1 item	540	25	7	1	75	1410	49
Crispy Chicken Sandwich	1 item	320	14	3	0	30	660	34
Black Forest Ham & Swiss Frescata	1 item	460	19	6	0	60	1770	50
Roasted Turkey & Swiss Frescata	1 item	470	20	6	0	60	150	51
Frescata Club	1 item	440	17	4	0	50	1600	49
Garden Sensations Salads & Fresh Fruit								
Creamy Ranch Dressing	2.25 oz.	230	23	4	0	15	580	NA
Spring Mix Salad w/o dressing or toppings	1 salad	180	11	6	0	30	220	NA
Honey Roasted Pecans	.75 oz.	130	13	2	0	0	65	NA
House Vinaigrette Dressing	2.25 oz.	190	18	3	0	0	750	NA